LIZ EARLE'S

Youthful Skin

GW00600709

LIZ EARLE'S

Youthful Skin

B⬛XTREE

Advice to the Reader

Before following any dietary advice contained in this book, it is recommended that you consult your doctor if you suffer from any health problems or special condition or are in any doubt.

First published in Great Britain in 1995 as *Liz Earle's Guide to Youthful Skin* by Boxtree Limited,
Broadwall House, 21 Broadwall, London SE1 9PL
This edition published in Great Britain in 1996 by Boxtree Limited

10 9 8 7 6 5 4 3 2 1

ISBN: 0 7522 0544 7

Text design by Blackjacks
Cover design by Slatter-Anderson

Printed and bound in Great Britain by
Mackays of Chatham PLC, Chatham, Kent

A CIP catalogue entry for this book is available from
the British Library

Contents

ACKNOWLEDGEMENTS

I am grateful to Sarah Purcell and Sarah Hamilton Fleming for helping to produce this book; also to Professor Nicholas Lowe MD, FRCP, FACP for his invaluable research and assistance. I am also grateful for market research figures provided by the Office of Population Censuses and Surveys, AGB Superpanel and MORI.

I am also indebted to the talented team at Boxtree, and to Rosemary Sandberg and Claire Bowles Publicity for their unfailing enthusiasm and support.

Introduction

In our youth-obsessed society it is no surprise that most of us want our skin to remain as youthful as possible. There are so many skincare and special treatments on offer it is difficult to know what to choose. Unfortunately, the cosmetic industry as a whole plays on our insecurities and is adept at advertising jars of miracle 'wrinkle removers'. But do any of these expensive skin treatments actually work? What is the best moisturiser? Can wrinkles really be held at bay? Can they be removed altogether?

I asked these questions and more when developing my own highly successful naturally active skincare range. As a result, this book has been written to give you the most up-to-date, honest and scientifically credible information on skin ageing. It reveals the ingredients that can delay fine lines and wrinkles, as well as the best strategy for a lifetime of youthful-looking skin.

Liz Earle

1

The Ageing Skin

As far back as 1935 *Vogue Magazine* told its readers 'No beauty can be a beauty today without good skin.' While the older model may currently be fashionable, we admire the likes of Lauren Hutton and Isabella Rossellini not for their beautiful wrinkles, but for their smooth, young-looking skin. Forget distinguished, nobody wants to look old and most of us long to look younger than our years.

The biggest compliment you can pay a women over the age of forty is to tell her she looks ten years younger than she is. Dr Martin Skinner, lecturer in psychology at the University of Warwick, explains: 'It is only when we are in our early teens that we try to look older. For most of their lives, people want to look youthful, because youthfulness is associated with vigour and good health.'

An opinion poll carried out by MORI (*Ageing – why fight it?*, October 1994) revealed that while for ageing men hair loss was considered the most worrying sign of getting older, for women aged thirty-five to forty-four, some 69 percent cited wrinkle-lined skin as being their main concern. Looking young in our society is seen as being linked with success. The same poll found that two out of three people believe a youthful appearance is important for success in job interviews, while slightly more said it was useful in terms of career prospects.

But an ageing population is a fact of life. The children of the baby boom are growing older. The number of sixteen to twenty-nine year old women will fall from 5.2m in 1992 to 4.3m by 2032, while the number of women aged sixty to seventy-four increase from 3.7m to 5.3m by 2032. Advertisers are beginning to change their tack to make sure we stay willing consumers of their products as we get older.

Anti-ageing creams are already one of the cosmetic market's success stories of this decade. British women spend more than £350 million on skincare products, of which over £100 million went on moisturisers alone, many of which now claim to prevent, delay or repair the signs of ageing. But in many cases, we're just buying hope in a jar, since any cream that says it can either stop your skin ageing or get rid of the wrinkles you already have could only do this by changing the actual structure of the skin. If it did this, then the cream would have to be classed as a drug rather than a cosmetic and you wouldn't be allowed to buy it. However, some naturally active skincare ingredients can help slow down the ageing process by protecting and nourishing the skin.

While skincare products, and moisturisers in particular, play an important role in keeping our skin looking young, there are more important factors to consider too. Our skin has its own chronological age, which may or may not be the same as our actual age – it can make us look ten years older or younger than we really are. The condition of our skin, including pore size and tanning ability, will depend mostly on the genes we inherit, which we can do nothing about. Take a look at the skin of your parents and grandparents – if their skin is prematurely lined, be warned that you will have to take extra care of yours.

Your skin type will also play a part. If you have oily skin, then wrinkles tend to appear later in life than in people with dry skin. Colour of skin is another factor – black skin usually weathers the years better than white because it is oilier and has a high level of in-built protection from harmful UV rays in the form of melanin, the pigment responsible for tanning. Black skin also seems to shed dead skin cells faster than white, keeping skin smoother and softer for longer.

Enemy number one of our skin is the sun. We now know that exposure to ultraviolet rays speeds up the ageing process as well as causing skin cancer. Other factors which will affect how our skin looks are the type of environment we live in, the kind of food we eat, and whether we smoke or drink.

What is Skin?

To have the youngest-looking complexion you can achieve, it is important to understand what skin is, how it works and what it needs to function at its best. No matter what colour, type or condition your skin, underneath the surface it all looks the same.

Skin is the largest organ in the body and its job is to protect our internal organs from the environment. It contains cells that are sensitive to touch, temperature and pain. It plays a vital role in keeping our body temperature constant through sweating when we get too hot and shivering when we're cold. Covering us from head to toe, the average adult's skin measures around 21 square feet (2m²) and weighs about 7lb, although it is never more than 4.7mm thick – the thickest areas of skin are found on the soles of our feet and our palms. The skin on our body is about 0.6mm thick, while that covering our face is much thinner, only 0.12mm, and the thinnest skin of all is found on our lips, which explains why they are so prone to cracking and splitting in cold weather. Each half-square inch of skin contains about ten hairs, 100 sweat glands, forty inches of blood vessels and fifteen sebaceous glands. Skin is a living organism which constantly renews itself, shedding dead cells all the time.

The Skin's Layers

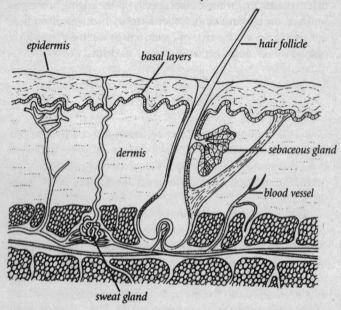

epidermis

basal layers

hair follicle

dermis

sebaceous gland

blood vessel

sweat gland

STRATUM CORNEUM

The layer of skin that you can see, the stratum corneum, is made up of dead skin cells which are gradually rubbed off and renewed by cells from underneath. We lose millions of these cells every day – if you were to look closely at household dust, it would be mainly made up of dead skin cells. This skin layer, about twenty cells thick, is completely renewed about once every four weeks. The new alpha-hydroxy acid (AHA) creams work by speeding up this process, revealing the softer, smoother skin beneath (see page 60).

The stratum corneum's function is to form a barrier from the outside world, stopping chemicals, dirt and germs from getting inside us. Any skincare products that you apply will act on this part. But while a moisturiser will improve the appearance of the stratum corneum and make it feel smoother and softer, it can only temporarily stick these dead cells back on to the skin. It provides a layer of moisture that helps keep the skin beneath hydrated, but only moisture taken from within can really improve its appearance over a longer period.

EPIDERMIS

Beneath the stratum corneum is the epidermis, a thin layer of four or five sheets of living cells. Its main function is to produce the keratin cells, a hard protein substance also found in hair and nails. The cells in the epidermis travel outwards, losing moisture in the process and becoming thinner and stiffer, eventually forming the new stratum corneum layer. The cells which produce the pigment called melanin are also found in the epidermis. Their function is to protect the lower layers from harmful ultraviolet rays. Exposure to strong sunlight encourages these cells to produce more pigment, which shows as a suntan. People with fair skin don't produce enough pigment to protect the lower layers, which is why skin cancer is more common in white-skinned people. It is also the reason why this type of skin ages more quickly than darker skin.

DERMIS

The deepest and thickest layer of skin is called the dermis, which provides the strength and structure of the skin. A thick, soft cushion of connective tissue lying beneath the epidermis, it determines the way our skin looks and behaves. The dermis can repair and renew itself, but does so much more slowly than the epidermis. As we age, the dermis naturally becomes thinner and weaker, causing skin to sag. Exposure to sunlight over the years speeds this process up, causing skin to lose its resilience and become wrinkled.

Collagen and elastin

The connective tissue which makes up the dermis is formed of collagen and elastin fibres. About 70 percent of this tissue is collagen, which can be divided into soluble (of which younger skin has more) and insoluble collagen. As we grow older, the ratio changes and we end up with more insoluble collagen, which is more easily broken down, thus resulting in drier, sagging skin. For women, in the ten years following the menopause, collagen levels fall by 30 percent as a result of oestrogen deficiency. You may have noticed that many skin creams contain collagen, which manufacturers claim will reinforce your own supplies. In fact, the collagen molecules used (extracted from cow skin) are much too large to penetrate the surface of the skin. The only way to put back the collagen your skin has lost is to inject it directly into the dermis (see page 79).

Elastin fibres make up about 5 percent of the dermis and are woven between strands of collagen to give extra strength and elasticity. As we age, elastin fibres lose their suppleness and skin becomes wrinkled and saggy. The best way to keep the skin fibres supple for longer is to provide the dermis with all the nutrients it needs to create collagen and elastin (see below).

Feeding the Skin

A network of blood vessels feeds the skin with the nutrients it needs to develop and repair itself. However, these nutrients can get redirected to other organs in the body, such as the heart or brain, leaving the skin underfed. A well-balanced diet will help ensure the skin gets the supplies it needs, while the best way to supplement it is with a daily dose of the essential fatty acids, vitamin E and lecithin. These can be found in cooking oils such as sunflower, corn and sesame seed and in supplements such as evening primrose oil.

Skin Through the Ages

Our facial skin is constantly changing and by the time we reach thirty, most of us have one or two lines, usually showing first around the eyes. While many women's skin starts to dry out, for others it can become oilier and they may even experience their first attack of acne. Our thirties can be a demanding time of life, with many of us juggling a career, family and home. The result is little time to spend on ourselves, with skin often neglected. But remember that all the time and effort we put in now will pay dividends later on.

Once we reach our forties, the signs of ageing become more obvious in the form of lines, wrinkles, broken veins and a generally less radiant complexion. Skin begins to dry out and using moisturiser daily becomes a more essential part of our daily skincare routine.

After the menopause the amount of oestrogen (known as the 'young' skin hormone) we produce slows down dramatically and the skin renews and repairs itself much more slowly, with the rate of cell replacement falling by half. The stratum corneum doesn't hold in moisture as well as it used to, oil gland activity slows down and the dermis becomes less resilient. The end result is drier, sagging skin. Many women find hormone replacement therapy (HRT) is useful at this time for its restorative effect on skin, as well as providing relief from other symptoms of the menopause.

Skin Ageing and Free Radicals

To survive, our body needs oxygen, which is then carried through the bloodstream to supply the living cells by a process called oxidation. But the process of converting oxygen into energy is flawed: a side-effect is the creation of free radicals. A free radical is an unstable molecule with an uneven number of electrons. Normally electrons are arranged in pairs, which gives them stability. The free radical will steal an electron from another molecule to even up its quota, but this creates another unstable molecule in the process.

A certain amount of free radicals are needed to kill off bacteria in the body, but too many of them causes problems. An excess upsets our normal cell activity, reacting with molecules and causing the damage which ultimately leads to a whole list of diseases including heart disease, some cancers, Parkinson's disease and rheumatoid arthritis. And while not immediately life threatening, scientists now believe that the action of free radicals on skin cells is a major cause of wrinkles and sagging skin.

Pollution, ultraviolet radiation from the sun and tobacco smoke all increase the levels of free radicals produced by the body. Free radicals harm the skin cells by destroying the membranes which surround them and encouraging collagen and elastin fibres to break down. Without the support these fibres provide, the skin starts to wrinkle and sag.

Antioxidant nutrients in the form of vitamins C, E and beta-carotene are the antidote to harmful free radicals. Beta-carotene and vitamin E help mop up the harmful free radicals while vitamin C also stimulates the cells that produce more collagen. Taking a daily supplement containing these three nutrients or eating foods which contain sufficient levels could keep wrinkles at bay for a little longer. We should also choose moisturisers that contain these vitamins to reinforce our skin's supplies directly.

The Three-Point Protection Plan

There is little we can do to stop the natural ravages of time on our skin, but here are three simple measures that everyone can take to keep it looking its best for as long as possible.

1. STAY OUT OF THE SUN

The skin's number one enemy is the sun. As well as causing skin cancer, dermatologists (skin specialists) believe exposure to sunlight is responsible for 90 percent of premature lines and wrinkles. So if the risk of cancer seems too slight to put you off getting a tan, think of the wrinkles you may be preventing instead!

While many dermatologists are sceptical about anti-ageing creams, they all agree that protecting your skin with a sunblock is the one measure that really works. No one is suggesting that we spend our life indoors or never take a foreign holiday, but there are sensible precautions we can take. 'Sun damage to skin cannot be reversed, but skin will repair itself to a small extent and further damage can be prevented,' says dermatologist and sun scientist Dr Anthony Young.

If you have fair skin, then you are more at risk from sun damage, but all skin types should protect themselves from strong sunlight. Dermatologists recommend that even black skin should be protected with a sunscreen with a sun protection factor of at least SPF4 (see page 28). Whereas UVB rays are known to cause skin to redden and burn, UVA rays are now believed to cause skin ageing. UVA rays are present throughout the year, so wear sun protection even in winter to be safe.

Take advice from the Australian slogan before you expose yourself: 'Slip on a T-shirt, slap on a hat and slop on sunscreen.'

2. ENRICH YOUR DIET WITH VITAMINS, OILS AND ANTIOXIDANTS

What you put inside your body is as important than anything you put on it. And when it comes to young-looking skin, beauty really does come from within. The food we eat has a big impact on our skin's condition and the way it ages, and no skin cream, no matter how expensive, can make up for a poor diet. To function properly our skin cells need plenty of vitamins and minerals, many of which can be found in food.

It is also important that we get enough fat in our diet in the form of unsaturated vegetable and fish oils. After all the bad reports fat has received in recent years, you could be forgiven for thinking you need to cut it out completely from your diet. But there are good and bad types of fat. Saturated fats should be eaten in moderation – we know that eating too much is a major cause of heart disease and also causes spotty, sallow-looking skin. These fats are derived from animal products and common examples are lard, milk, cream, butter and eggs. The good fats are polyunsaturated and monounsaturated fats, derived mainly from vegetables and plants. Examples include olive oil, sunflower oil, walnut oil and sesame oil. Fish oils are also very good for you. Essential fatty acids (found in polyunsaturated fats) are vital for healthy skin cells, keeping them moist and strong. They encourage the production of strong collagen and elastin fibres in the dermis, helping prevent wrinkling and sagging.

The most important vitamins for healthy skin are A, C and E.

* Beta-carotene, found in brightly coloured vegetables and fruits, is converted by the body into vitamin A as it needs it. Vitamin A is important for keeping skin tissue healthy and helps prevent dryness and flaking.

* Vitamin C plays an important role in the production of collagen, which keeps skin smooth and supple. The best sources are citrus fruits and fresh vegetables. In winter when fresh produce is less readily available, taking a daily vitamin C supplement is a good idea.

* Vitamin E, found in many face creams, can help rehydrate dry skin. The best source is wheatgerm oil, while

other good sources are sunflower seeds, almonds, eggs and wholemeal bread.

Other healthy-skin supplements include evening primrose oil and borage oil which both contain high levels of gamma-linolenic acid (GLA), an essential fatty acid which has been found to strengthen skin cells and increase their moisture level.

3. FOLLOW AN EFFECTIVE SKINCARE ROUTINE

Cleansing and moisturising are the key to an effective skincare routine, although they cannot undo damage caused by the sun or a poor diet. When combined with a good diet and a sensible attitude to sunbathing, an effective skincare routine is the icing on the cake.

The products you use do not have to be expensive or state of the art, but you may need to experiment a little before you find what suits you. Avoid using soap and water on your face as soap is highly alkaline and can upset the skin's natural acidic protective film; nor can it cleanse the pores thoroughly enough. For most skins, an oil-based cleanser is best, used morning and evening.

The job of a moisturiser is to keep water in the stratum corneum or outer layer of skin. It doesn't matter which type you choose, as long as it feels comfortable on your skin. As a general rule, apply twice daily after cleansing.

A water spray or a spray-on tonic is useful for topping up your skin's moisture level throughout the day, especially if you live or work in a dry environment.

Although not essential, weekly exfoliation helps improve the texture of your skin by sloughing off the dead skin cells that can make it appear dull, dry and flaky. See page 70 for some home-made recipes. You can achieve the same effect by gently buffing the skin with a soft muslin cloth.

——2——

The Sun Factor

Designer Coco Chanel has a lot to answer for. Apart from her famous Chanel suits and bags, copied throughout the world, she also sparked off another twentieth-century trend – the suntan. When she stepped off the Duke of Westminster's yacht after a cruise, in the early 1930s, sporting a golden-brown tan, a new age of modern sun worship was born. The fashionable set flocked to resorts such as St Tropez to fry themselves golden brown, the sign of a wealthy, leisured life. The trend continued, peaking in the Sixties and Seventies when air travel and holiday prices became more affordable and sunshine was just an hour's flight away.

Sun damage takes years to accumulate, and it wasn't until the Eighties that a rising number of skin cancer cases caused dermatologists to ask serious questions about the danger of too much exposure to the sun. The conclusion they came to was that our passion for toasting our pale northern skins at every opportunity was to blame.

Some 40,000 new cases of skin cancer are diagnosed in this country every year. The good news is that 95 percent of these cases are the less serious, curable types. But malignant melanoma, the serious and potentially fatal skin cancer, is now the most rapidly increasing cancer in Britain, with about 4,000 new cases each year, double what it was ten years ago. Among women it is now the third most common cancer. Melanoma favours fair-skinned people living in hot countries, which is why Australia has such a high rate. Getting badly sunburnt in child-hood is also thought to be an important factor, and by the age of twenty we have built up half our lifetime's sun exposure. According to leading American dermatologist Dr Karen Burke, if a child is properly protected from the sun until the age of ten, the chances of developing skin cancer in later life are reduced by 80 percent. So remember always to protect children from the sun – they'll thank you for it in years to come.

According to Dr John Hawk, consultant dermatologist at St John's Institute of Dermatology, St Thomas' Hospital, 'The only safe tan is the one you were born with. Any sort of acquired tan is always associated with damage.' However, if you spent a lot of time in the sun as a child and remember getting sunburnt, don't panic. It doesn't necessarily mean that you will develop skin cancer, but it should serve as a warning to take extra care from now on.

While the dark side of the sun is skin cancer, sunlight is now also believed to be the cause of 90 percent of wrinkles, according to Dr Hawk. The fact that people today live much longer than they used to also plays a part – their skin is exposed to the sun for many more years than in previous centuries, even if they do protect it properly. But compare a nun's face to that of a Mediterranean farmer, or feel the skin on your inner arm compared with the back of your hand and you will get the picture: sun is bad news for skin. 'My advice to anyone wanting to keep their skin looking younger for longer is to stop sunbathing and stay off sunbeds,' says Dr Hawk.

When Sun Meets Skin

Sunlight reaching the skin consists of visible light, infrared rays and ultraviolet rays. The important part where skin is concerned is ultraviolet rays, which are divided into long, medium and short wavebands – UVA, UVB and UVC respectively.

* UVC rays are absorbed by the ozone layer in the stratosphere before they reach earth, and there is no evidence yet to suggest that any filter through.

* UVB rays are by far the most damaging, being responsible for skin cancer, although making up only 20 percent of ultraviolet radiation. These rays are absorbed by the epidermis and the upper layers of the dermis, stimulating the production of melanin which gives us our tan; UVB rays also help synthesise vitamin D in the body. If our skin is exposed to them for too long it reddens and burns. UVB rays are present whenever the sun shines and are four times more prevalent in summer than winter between the hours of 11am and 3pm, which is why we should stay out of the midday sun. However, the hole in the ozone layer means that more UVB rays are getting through and some experts believe that for every 1 percent fall in ozone there is a 2 percent increase in UV levels reaching the earth, resulting in a 3 percent increase in skin cancers.

* UVA rays make up 80 percent of ultraviolet radiation and the damage they cause is less apparent. These rays penetrate deep into the dermis and over time they damage the collagen and elastin fibres which give skin its support, leading to what dermatologists call photo-ageing, or wrinkling. UVA rays are responsible for sun-induced allergies such as prickly heat and help generate the harmful free radicals. UVA rays are present all year round, even in cloudy weather, which is why you should *always* wear sun protection. UVA rays are also emitted from sunbeds so, while most tanning machines won't burn, they will accelerate the ageing process within the skin.

How the Sun Ages the Skin

When sunlight hits our skin, complex changes take place below the surface. In the epidermis, the pigment-producing cells called melanocytes produce melanin, or what we refer to as a suntan. So that golden-brown colour we so long for is actually a sign of skin damage. As a reaction to this, the stratum corneum thickens in an attempt to stop more harmful rays getting through. The darker the tan, the more damage is being done to the skin.

While UVB rays trigger the tanning action, they also encourage the development of freckles, uneven patches of pigment and 'liver spots', usually on the face and backs of hands. These can appear as early as the age of thirty and once we have them they are difficult to get rid of.

UVA rays penetrate much deeper into the skin, reaching the dermis. The damage they cause is two-fold: they destroy the supporting network of collagen and elastin fibres, which eventually leads to wrinkling. In addition they cause free-radical,damage, which changes the cell's DNA (their genetic blueprint) and so the cell loses the ability to repair itself. This is now believed to be a major factor in skin ageing.

Wrinkling is only seen on sun-exposed parts of the body, usually the face, neck and hands. The more time we spend in the sun, the more wrinkled our skin will become. Darker skins are much less prone to wrinkling because the high level of natural melanin pigment that they contain is a protective filter to the UV rays.

Sunscreens

'A sunscreen is the best anti-ageing product available; the best and the most proven,' says Mitch Wortzman, president of dermatology for skincare company Neutrogena in Los Angeles.

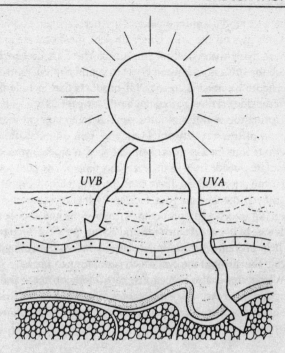

Whether you want to prevent damage or avoid further harm to your skin, the message is clear: use a sunscreen on your face and neck every day, rain or shine. Most ultraviolet rays can penetrate through clouds, water and even glass.

You may think that most days you're not at risk from sun damage, but those few minutes that you spend walking to your car, waiting for the bus, going out at lunchtime, or even when in your car, as a small amount of the UV rays can penetrate the windscreen, all add up to cumulative sun damage over the years. Many moisturisers and foundations now include sunscreens, but they can irritate sensitive skins. Always remember to look on the label to make sure it offers UVA and UVB protection. The safest forms of sunscreen are reflective barriers, such as finely ground titanium dioxide. This inert substance bounces the sun's rays off the skin. Unfortunately, most suncare products are made with chemical sun filters. These are designed to absorb the sun's rays, but can cause irritation and skin sensitivity. The best answer is to look for products that include titanium dioxide on their ingredient label (see page 29).

During the summer months you'll need to take extra care. Stay out of the sun between 11am and 3pm on hot days and never put your face in direct sunlight. Try to arrange your day so you are outside only in the early morning or late afternoon. When you are outside in direct sunlight, wear a broad-brimmed hat to keep the sun off your face and a high protection sunscreen. Sit under a sun umbrella when possible and choose the shady side of the street when out and about. Wearing sunglasses will help prevent cataracts in later life as well as protecting the delicate skin around the eye, which is so prone to ageing.

Winter sun is also dangerous, particularly on snow and in mountainous areas, where the glare is reflected directly back at you. So just because it feels cold, don't be fooled, you still need high protection on your face.

ANTIOXIDANTS

Free-radical damage is partly activated by sunlight, but nature provides an antidote in the form of antioxidant vitamins A (in the form of beta-carotene), C, and E. Take them daily in your diet and choose skincare products that contain them.

Many creams contain vitamin E, the most effective solution to sun-induced free-radical activity (see page 34). Taking a daily dose of 400iu (international units) vitamin E can help protect skin from sun damage – according to a report by dermatologist Dr Karen Burke, it has the same effect as having a sunscreen of SPF4 on your skin. Dermatologist Dr John Hawk points out that, although antioxidants can't prevent sun damage, 'free radicals account for about 10 percent of sun damage to the skin, so by protecting yourself from them you can reduce some of the harm.'

CHOOSING A SUNSCREEN

If you're going to spend long spells out in a hot sun, then a sunscreen is a must. But when it comes to choosing one, the scientific terms can be confusing. The first thing you'll notice on the bottle is the letters 'SPF' (sun protection factor) followed by a number. An SPF is there to tell you how long you can safely stay in the sun without burning. For example, if your bare skin normally reddens after ten minutes in the sun, using a product with SPF8 will allow you to stay out for eighty minutes without burning (10 x 8 = 80). But this will vary from person to person – the paler your skin, the quicker you will burn and the higher SPF protection you will need to be safe.

WHICH SPF DO I NEED?

Dermatologists divide skin types into six groups, with group one being the fairest and six the darkest. To work out which SPF you need, first decide which skin type you are.

* **Type 1:** Your skin is naturally very pale, with a fine texture and a translucent quality. It freckles easily and always burns in strong sun. It probably reddens within ten minutes of unprotected exposure to sunlight. Your skin never develops a proper tan, and peels after burning. People with this skin type often have fair or red hair and blue or green eyes.

* **Type 2:** Your skin is naturally fair and tends to freckle. When exposed to strong sun you burn in about twenty minutes. Your skin does tan, but with difficulty. This is probably the most common skin type in the UK, with most having fair hair and blue eyes.

* **Type 3:** Your skin is medium toned, not really olive but not fair either. You don't usually freckle and your skin tans fairly easily and doesn't usually burn. Your hair is generally dark and your eyes brown.

* **Type 4:** Your skin is olive in tone – the typical Mediterranean look. It doesn't freckle, tans easily and doesn't often burn. But don't be fooled into thinking it doesn't need protection – the ageing UVA rays still penetrate deep into the dermis if you don't protect it. Hair is usually dark and eyes brown.

* **Type 5:** Your skin is naturally brown, typically Asian, Indian, north African or Arabic in origin. Your skin almost never burns and darkens quickly on exposure to sun. Some sun protection is still recommended to guard against wrinkling.

* **Type 6:** Yours is the darkest skin tone, dark brown or black, typically African or West Indian in origin. You never burn and skin darkens quickly on sun exposure. Dermatologists still recommend you protect yourself in strong sunlight.

CHOOSING AN SPF FOR YOUR SKIN TYPE

The level of protection your skin needs will depend on the time of year, whether you're at home or on holiday, and how long you spend outside. Check the SPF chart to see which SPF you need.

WRITTEN IN THE STARS

Always choose a sunscreen that offers UVA as well as UVB protection. To check the level of UVA screening in a product, Boots has introduced a star rating system which is now featured on major suncare brands. Look at the back of the pack where you

MODERATE

GOOD

SUPERIOR

MAXIMUM

will see a number of stars, ranging from one to four. These stars tell you how much UVA protection there is in relation to the UVB protection given. Levels range from one star (minimum) to four stars (maximum). However, these symbols only represent a ratio – an SPF15 product may only have one star, but it will give more protection against UVA rays than an SPF4 product with four stars. It is confusing, but to be safe, opt for a product with a high factor with maximum star rating.

WHAT'S IN A SUNSCREEN?

A sunscreen is either physical or chemical in action. The physical type is based on powdered minerals such as titanium dioxide, zinc oxide and ferric oxide and works by forming a physical barrier against the sun that reflects or scatters the sun's rays. Safest for use on sensitive skins, they are effective at blocking UVA and UVB rays. While the downside of these ingredients used to be that they left a chalky white residue on the skin, scientists can now break down titanium dioxide into much smaller particles by a process called micronisation, making them much less visible and more versatile. They are now used in

SUN PROTECTION FACTOR CHART						
	SPFs for skin type					
	1	2	3	4	5	6
UK/North Europe	10–15	10–12	8–10	6–8	6	4–6
Mediterranean	15–20	12–15	10–12	8–10	6–8	6
Tropics/Africa	20–30	15–25	12–20	10–15	8–10	6–8

common ones are PABA (B-vitamin para-aminobenzoic acid), Padimate O, cinnamates, homosalate and octyl salicylate. Their disadvantage is the risk of skin irritation, so look for PABA-free sunscreens and avoid chemical sunscreens on the face.

Plant oils such as sesame oil also offer natural protection and are often included in sunscreens as they soften skin too. Many brands now include vitamin A and E to help prevent free-radical damage, or a synthetically produced version of melanin for extra protection.

FACE-SAVING TIPS

* If in doubt, choose a higher factor sunscreen than you think you need. You can never have too much protection.

* Apply sunscreen liberally. If you're too thrifty with it you'll lower the effectiveness of the product, ending up with SPF8 instead of SPF10, for example.

* Apply sunscreen to your skin thirty minutes before going outside to give it a chance to get working.

* In strong sun reapply sunscreen every two hours. At the beach or pool, choose a waterproof formulation and reapply after every swim.

* Buying a high-factor sunscreen doesn't mean you can safely expose your skin to hot sun all day. You should still limit your exposure time depending on the SPF of your sunscreen and *always* avoid the sun between 11am and 3pm.

* If you're playing sports in the sun, use a waterproof or sweat-resistant product.

* Remember that water and snow intensify the effects of the sun, reflecting the ultraviolet rays back at you.

* *Never* expose your face to direct sunlight. Protect it every day with a sunscreen and with a sunblock in strong sun to prevent premature ageing.

DAILY PROTECTION ROUTINE

Of course, you'll need a different level of protection depending on the time of year and how much time you spend in the sun. During autumn and winter, when you're only outside for short periods, a product with SPF5 should be sufficient. During summer, most dermatologists recommend we switch to SPF15.

Get into the habit of applying some sun protection cream containing UVA and UVB filters on top of your daily moisuriser. Don't forget your neck – a smooth face with a wrinkly neck will not look attractive! If you wear foundation you can increase your protection further by choosing one with sun filters. A layer of powder gives a further top-up, since all make-up contains powdered particles that help block out ultraviolet rays. Lips are vulnerable too, so wearing a lipstick or lip balm with sunscreen will help protect them and keep them soft.

The Truth about Sunbeds

Many people mistakenly believe that using a sunlamp or sunbed will give them a quicker and safer tan without burning. While sunbeds now only emit UVA rays, these are present in higher levels than are found in natural sunlight. These rays penetrate deep into the dermis, destroying the supporting fibres and leading to premature wrinkling and sagging of the skin.

Sunbeds can also cause allergic reactions such as rashes and itching in sensitive skin.

Dermatologist Dr John Hawk says: 'While one or two sunbeds probably won't have done much harm, if you use them regularly the damage to your skin will slowly build up.' If this isn't enough to discourage you, doctors have now proved links between skin cancer and the use of sunbeds, and guidelines on their use have been revised as a result. But in terms of youthful skin the best advice of all is to steer clear of sunbeds altogether.

Repairing Sun-Damaged Skin

While dermatologists always used to say that sun-damaged skin was beyond repair, new evidence suggests this is no longer the case. President of dermatology at Neutrogena Mitch Wortzman says: 'The evidence says that skin can repair itself as part of a natural process by avoiding further sun exposure. This has been proven in the US in nursing homes, where old people who led previously active, outdoor lives start to lead a more secluded existence. The skin starts to repair the sun damage on its own.'

But it seems there is only so much the skin can do to help itself. Once the DNA (the blueprint for reproducing new cells) inside the cell has been badly damaged, nothing can help it.

Products which help to repair photo-aged skin all work on the principle of speeding up the rate at which the cells renew themselves. The most widely known anti-ageing 'cure' is tretinoin, or retinoic acid (marketed as Retin-A), a synthetic form of vitamin A. Originally prescribed for acne treatment in the 1970s, patients found that it not only helped their spots, but their skin looked smoother and less wrinkled too. Scientists discovered that the skin cells were renewing themselves more quickly, which led to a faster turnover on the skin's surface, and that collagen and elastin production was boosted too.

A study on the restoration of collagen production in sun-damaged skin by use of retinoic acid, published in the *New England Journal of Medicine* (1993, no.329), concluded that 'the formation of collagen 1 is significantly decreased in photo-damaged human skin, and this process is partly restored by treatment with tretinoin'. A lack of collagen in the dermis has been directly linked to the appearance of wrinkles and 'although tretinoin can directly induce collagen synthesis it can also decrease the breakdown of collagen by inducing tissue inhibitors of collagenese,' says the report. It seems that this combination of preventing the existing collagen from breaking down while stimulating the body to produce more is the key to its success.

But it's not all good news. To be effective, retinoic acid has to be used in a high concentration (usually 0.1 percent), which causes skin to redden, inflame and peel. Once retinoic acid has been used, the skin becomes hyper-sensitive to sunlight and a sunblock must be worn at all times. Also, as Dr John Hawk says, 'Retin-A has been claimed by many as an anti-ageing substance as it changes the way in which skin grows. But even this cannot repair DNA damage.' The possibility of an increased risk of getting skin cancer has not yet been ruled out. Scientists are researching the use of new, less harmful forms of retinoic acid.

A newer anti-ageing treatment is the alpha-hydroxy acids (AHAs), which are naturally present in fruit, milk and sugar cane. These work by encouraging the skin to shed its top layer more quickly by softening the cement that holds the cells together, revealing the smoother, younger skin underneath. Studies have shown that fine lines and wrinkles may be reduced after two to six months of use. But to be effective you need fairly high levels of the AHAs, which can irritate sensitive skin – most sensitive-skin brands will not include AHA products in their ranges for this reason. Look for a minimum level of 1 percent in any AHA product you buy – any less and it won't do any good;

but much more and it may cause irritation, so it is up to you to see if these products suit your skin.

The antioxidant vitamin E is good for repairing sunburnt or sun-damaged skin as it helps curb free-radical activity. Present in high quantities in wheatgerm oil, you can use this directly on sunburnt skin to help repair the damage. Look for the natural form of vitamin E in any aftersun cream that you buy (see page 43).

3

The Anti-Ageing Diet

Effective skincare is important, but no matter what care we lavish on our skin from the outside, it can never make up for what we feed it on the inside. An expensive moisturiser or facial treatment won't cancel out the effects of a poor diet. Our skin cells, just like any other cell in our body, rely on a constant supply of nourishment to survive and develop. The only real way to improve the condition of our skin and keep it looking younger for longer is to feed it with a well-balanced diet, rich in vitamins, minerals and other useful nutrients.

Looking at our face reveals more about our health than you'd imagine. Dark shadows under the eyes not only signify tiredness but also tension, and puffiness is a sign of liver and kidney problems. Spots indicate a poor diet or a sluggish lymphatic system, while rashes are due to allergies, internal imbalances and stress. Tiny red veins on the cheeks and round the nose are the result of too much caffeine, alcohol, sugar and spices or exposure to extremes in temperature. A dry, flaking skin indicates deficiencies in vitamin E and essential fatty acids. For a glowing, healthy and young-looking complexion we need to treat our skin as part of our body as a whole, not as a separate entity.

The skin is fed by a rich network of blood vessels which keep it supplied with essential nutrients to stay healthy. But these nutrients are not always directed to the skin – other organs in the body may take priority, leaving the skin malnourished. To ensure this doesn't happen, we need to eat a well-balanced diet every day, swapping high levels of saturated fat, sugar and additives for fresh foods prepared with the minimum of processing.

Skin Enemies

While eating a healthy diet is important, continuing with bad habits can undo your good work, cancelling out the beneficial effects of many of the vitamins and minerals we eat. So before you embark on your healthy-skin plan, make sure you know the skin enemies so you can avoid them.

* Smoking just half a packet of cigarettes a day for two years can double your number of premature wrinkles, according to American research. Smoking activates harmful free radicals, destroys vitamin C and starves the cells of oxygen. It weakens the collagen and elastin fibres, causing sagging and wrinkling. According to research by American dermatologist Dr Karen Burke, smokers aged forty could have the same number of wrinkles as a sixty-year-old, with particularly prominent ones around the eyes and lips. Skin becomes thinner when you smoke, the complexion has an ashen, gaunt appearance and there are more broken veins. And remember that the effects of passive smoking will be similar, so aim to live and work in a smoke-free environment.

* While a glass of red wine a day may be beneficial, having a protective effect on heart and the cardiovascular system due to its antioxidant ingredients, any more than this is harmful. Alcohol dehydrates the body, stripping cells of vital moisture and causing premature ageing. Drinking depletes nutrients, in particular vitamins A, B, C, magnesium, zinc and the essential fatty acids. The occasional drink is fine, but don't overdo it!

* Caffeine, found in coffee, tea, cola-based fizzy drinks and chocolate, depletes some vitamins and minerals as

well as increasing the risk of health problems such as high blood pressure, insomnia and headaches. A highly addictive drug: about 60mg of caffeine are contained in each cup of coffee. Coffee also contains a toxic substance called benzoic acid, which cannot be eliminated by the kidneys until converted into hippuric acid by an amino acid called glycine. This amino acid is found in collagen as well as the liver, and the body diverts it from collagen in order to get rid of toxins, depleting our collagen levels. This may have an adverse effect on the structure of our skin.

* Saturated animal fat (fatty meat, lard, suet and cheese) is one of the main causes of heart disease, clogging up the arteries and slowing down our lymphatic system which gets rid of toxins in the body. A sluggish flow of lymph shows up as spots, dull skin, cellulite and scalp problems.

* Most of us consume too much salt. The World Health Organisation recommends a maximum of 1/8oz per day, while most of us eat around 1/2oz – more for those who add extra salt to their food. Too much salt overloads the kidneys, preventing them from filtering fluids properly and leading to fluid retention. It can cause bags under the eyes and cellulite on hips and thighs.

* In Britain we are notorious for the large amounts of sugary foods we eat, with the average person consuming a huge 1kg per week. Sugar is high in calories, causing weight gain, while containing no nourishment at all. It has been linked to skin disorders such as acne, lowered immunity, kidney damage and diabetes as well as tooth decay. Sugar substitutes such as honey, fructose and

molasses are not much better, while chemically produced saccharin has been linked with cancer. The answer is to try to wean yourself off very sweet foods gradually, until you can cut them out of your diet altogether.

✱ Over-eating, particularly of highly processed foods and animal proteins, can age you. Women with young-looking skin usually consume fewer calories but eat a diet rich in fresh fruits and vegetables and low in saturated fat. Eating more than your body needs increases the production of toxins and encourages a build-up of waste matter within the system. Aim to eat less, but more healthily.

✱ While eating too much does your skin no good, constant dieting will result in dried-out skin which is more prone to premature ageing. Most diets are low in fat, and not enough fat causes a dull complexion because the cells are being deprived of essential moisture. Enough of the right kind of fats (the essential fatty acids) is vital for youthful, healthy, 'springy' skin (see page 46 for more details on fats).

The Vitamins Your Skin Needs and Where to Find Them

VITAMIN A

Think of this as the anti-ageing vitamin as it is essential for skin repair, protection and growth. In the vegetable form of beta-carotene, this important antioxidant helps fight the effects of damaging free-radical activity in our skin cells. Vitamin A helps keep the skin elastic. Not enough vitamin A will result in dull, flaky skin and premature wrinkles.

Vitamin A can be divided into two types, beta-carotene and retinol. Beta-carotene is converted by the body into vitamin A as needed, while the rest is used as an antioxidant. It is found in highest quantities in brightly coloured vegetables and fruit such as carrots, peppers, oranges, broccoli, spinach and apricots. By acting as an antioxidant it helps prevent the facial lines that are a result of free-radical damage. It can also protect the skin from the ageing effects of sun damage and it is worth taking extra beta-carotene supplements before a tropical holiday. The best form of beta-carotene is a natural source, extracted from a nutritious algae, found in good-quality skin supplements.

Retinol is found in animal produce such as eggs, milk, cheese, butter, liver and oily fish such as salmon. While a certain amount is important, an excess of retinol can be dangerous, particularly in pregnant women, who are now advised against eating liver, a particularly rich source.

VITAMIN B

There are some dozen or so vitamins in the B-complex family and they are all important in keeping our skin healthy and for maintaining our immune system. Vitamin B2, or riboflavin, plays an important role in the transportation of oxygen to the skin cells. It is found in dairy products, yeast, liver, wheatgerm and leafy vegetables. A lack of vitamin B2 results in a slower regeneration of skin cells, which eventually shows up as dry, wrinkled skin, cracked lips, hair loss and whiteheads.

B3, or niacin, helps the body to break down fats and is important for healthy skin tissue. Found in yeast, nuts, chicken, oily fish and dried fruit, a deficiency results in rough, flaky skin.

B5 is thought to have an anti-ageing, strengthening effect on skin when combined with antioxidants. It is found in yeast, liver, nuts, eggs, wheatgerm and wheat bran and it is also available in the form of pantothenic acid or calcium pantothenate in the better skin supplements.

B6, or pyridoxine, is known as an anti-stress vitamin and is important in cell oxidation and tissue repair and growth. Also thought to improve the symptoms of premenstrual syndrome (PMS), low levels can lead to both dry and oily skin, dandruff and rashes. Vitamin B6 can be depleted by the hormone oestrogen, so if you take the contraceptive pill or are on HRT (hormone replacement therapy) you may need to increase your intake. The best sources are wheatgerm, bananas, nuts, oily fish, brown rice and vegetables.

Biotin, a B-complex vitamin, can help improve skin condition. A deficiency may show up as dermatitis. Good sources include oily fish, corn, brown rice, yeast and eggs. Again, good-quality skin supplements should contain biotin.

Choline, another B-complex vitamin, is also important in helping the skin cells to repair and renew themselves, keeping skin looking young. Best sources are lecithin (see page 48), steak, eggs, nuts, pulses, citrus fruits and leafy vegetables.

VITAMIN C

Vitamin C, or ascorbic acid, is one of the best-known and most important vitamins for healthy skin, as well as having a host of other uses. It is responsible for producing the protein collagen, which supports the structure of the skin. Vitamin C is also one of the essential antioxidants that act against the formation of harmful free radicals which are a major cause of premature ageing. It is water soluble and travels through the fluid between the cells, fighting off free radicals as they are formed.

Smoking a single cigarette is thought to knock out 25mg of vitamin C from the body, so it is particularly important for smokers to increase their intake of this vitamin.

We all know that vitamin C is found in citrus fruits, particularly oranges and blackcurrants, but it is easily destroyed by cooking, pollution and alcohol. It is not stored in the body, so we need to consume foods containing vitamin C every day. Best sources are all citrus fruits, acerola cherries, blackcurrants, strawberries, green peppers, broccoli, Brussels sprouts and potatoes. Premium skincare ranges and skin supplements should contain high levels of vitamin C for inside-out protection.

Foods rich in vitamin C also contain bioflavonoids, a group of colouring pigments that help protect the fruit or vegetable against damage from oxidation. These bioflavonoids are important for the skin as they work together with vitamin C to strengthen the blood capillaries, prevent bruising and ward off infection. Good sources are citrus fruit skins, lemon juice, apricots, cherries, green peppers, tomatoes and grapes. One of the most useful bioflavonoids is rutin, which helps strengthen the capillary walls of tiny facial blood vessels. Rutin is often found listed as a separate ingredient in skincare supplements.

VITAMIN E

Vitamin E, or tocopherol, is the skin's saviour. Probably the most important antioxidant, it fights off free-radical activity and protects our skin from the signs of premature ageing. It also ensures better use of oxygen by the skin cells. Scientists believe that taking around 50mg of natural vitamin E every day can help repair sun-damaged skin and decrease your chances of getting skin cancer. Too little vitamin E results in muscle weakness and the loss of red blood cells. Vitamin E works in tandem with selenium (see page 44) to neutralise free radicals, so it's important to take sufficient quantities of both.

The best sources of vitamin E are wholegrains, particularly wheatgerm, unrefined vegetable oils such as wheatgerm, sunflower and safflower, sunflower seeds, eggs, cod liver oil, peanuts and brown rice. Vitamin E levels are depleted by food refining, cooking and storage. Its action can also be inhibited by the oestrogen in the contraceptive pill and HRT (hormone replacement therapy).

VITAMINS FOR HEALTHY SKIN

Vitamin	Source	Action
A (retinol)	Dairy products, liver, cod liver oil	Aids elasticity, prevents dryness
A (beta-carotene)	Brightly coloured fruit and vegetables	Antioxidant, protects from sun damage and premature ageing
B2 (riboflavin)	Dairy products, yeast, liver, wheatgerm, leafy vegetables	Aids skin repair, transports oxygen to cells
B3 (niacin)	Yeast, chicken, oily fish, cheese, dried fruit	Keeps tissue healthy, improves skin condition
B5 (pantothenic acid)	Yeast, liver, nuts, wheatgerm, eggs	Anti-ageing, skin strengthener
B6 (pyridoxine)	Brewer's yeast, wheatgerm, oatflakes, bananas, oily fish, brown rice, vegetables	Aids tissue repair and growth
C (ascorbic acid)	Acerola cherries, blackcurrants, citrus fruits, green peppers	Antioxidant, aids collagen and connective tissue production
E (tocopherol)	Wheatgerm, unrefined vegetable oils, peanuts, eggs, brown rice	Antioxidant, aids skin repair, protects from premature ageing

In the western world, it is hard to obtain high levels of vitamin E in the diet. Anyone concerned about ageing skin should certainly consider a supplement containing at least 50mg of vitamin E. Make sure the vitamin E is from a natural source, not synthetically produced, as this is much less effective. Natural vitamin E will be listed as 'd-alpha-tocopherol' while the synthetic type is called 'dl-alpha-tocopherol'.

Minerals and Trace Elements for Healthy Skin

Needed only in tiny amounts to do their job, these are essential for keeping skin healthy. Some of the most important ones include:

Copper. Important for creating the skin pigment melanin and connective tissue, it is contained in collagen and elastin and helps give smooth, clear skin. With antioxidant properties, it helps fight premature ageing. Good sources include liver, seafood, nuts, lentils, oats and rye.

Magnesium. Working with the B vitamins and essential fatty acids, it helps repair and maintain skin cells. Good sources are nuts, sesame seeds, brown rice, seafood, bananas and wholemeal flour.

Manganese. This helps build the connective tissue that supports the skin. It also plays a role in the creation of glycoproteins, a combination of glucose and protein which forms a protective coating around the cells to help ward off free-radical attacks. Best sources are wholegrains, green leafy vegetables, wholemeal bread, avocados and pineapples.

Selenium. Important for keeping skin tissue strong and healthy, it works with vitamin E as another antioxidant in scavenging free radicals. It helps to keep skin supple by preventing the oxidation of polyunsaturated fatty acids which weakens cell membranes. Research suggests that it may work as an anti-cancer agent too. Best sources are fish, seafood, meat, whole grains, cereals and dairy products. Because it is taken up by the food chain, it can be depleted by the poor quality of the soil in which the food you eat is grown.

Silicon. Also known as silica, this is present in tiny quantities in connective tissue. Silicon is important for healthy skin, keeping it supple and strong. The best sources are organically grown produce, particularly vegetables. Silica supplements are especially useful for maintaining skin elasticity.

Sulphur. Often neglected, this trace element helps build protein tissue in the body. It is needed to create the keratin found in skin cells as well as the hair and nails. The best sources are shellfish, horseradish, kidney beans and peas.

Zinc. Also an antioxidant, zinc is found in tissues throughout the body and is an important part of the DNA that gives life to cells. It aids in the production of some eighty enzymes and hormones in the body. Important for a clear, healthy complexion, zinc promotes skin repair, strengthens elastin and collagen fibres and helps to improve skin problems such as acne, and skin texture and tone. Sources include meat, nuts, wholegrains, seafood, sardines and eggs. It can be depleted by alcohol and drugs such as aspirin and the contraceptive pill.

Echinacea

A herbal extract which has been proven to stimulate the immune system. A member of the coneflower family, which grows in North America, echinacea has long been used in traditional remedies for fighting off infection. It works by stimulating the white blood cells, increasing their number and activity. As a skincare aid it is believed to stimulate the regeneration of connective tissue and epidermal cells and accelerate the healing process. Many vitamins and minerals have been found in the echinacea plant, including vitamin C, essential fatty acids, linoleic acid and polysaccharides, which promote wound healing. There are some nine varieties of echinacea, and those commonly used in high-quality skincare supplements are *Echinacea purpurea* (so called because of its dark purple flowers), which contains high levels of polysaccharides, and *Echinacea angustifolia*.

Alfalfa

These seeds, when sprouted, are a good, inexpensive way to feed your skin with a wealth of nutrients. The sprouts are best eaten shortly after germination when they measure 1–5cm long. Alfalfa is one of the best dietary sources of chlorophyll, which is essential for wound repair. They are also a good source of protein, containing all eight essential amino acids, vitamins, minerals and several enzymes which improve digestion. Alfalfa is a particularly good source of calcium and the B vitamins including vitamin B12, which together promote healthy skin. Alfalfa seeds can be bought already sprouted or it is easy to sprout them yourself at home. First rinse the seeds, then put them in a glass jar, covering it with a piece of muslin or kitchen towel, and secure with a rubber band. Rinse the seeds at least twice a day, leaving the jar on its side to drain. After approximately three days your jar should contain tasty, nutritious alfalfa sprouts which make a delicious addition to salads and sandwiches. Because of the wealth of amino acids and nutrients it contains, alfalfa seed extract may also be found in supplements to strengthen the skin.

Kelp

This variety of seaweed is a rich source of iodine which speeds up the metabolism and maintains a steady rate of detoxification. In the past, we would have obtained sufficient amounts of iodine through our foods from the soil, but modern farming methods have depleted the soil of many important trace elements. Our bodies need to detox regularly, especially in the polluted atmosphere in which many of us live. If we eat an unhealthy diet, smoke cigarettes or drink alcohol, our systems can soon become clogged up with waste and this is often reflected in the condition of our skin. Good skin supplements often contain kelp to encourage our bodies to eliminate waste, helping to create a clearer complexion.

The Role of Essential Fatty Acids

With a largely undeserved reputation as the cause of spots and greasy skin, fats are vital for improving skin health and keeping those wrinkles at bay. But there are good and bad fats. Saturated animal fats are the type to be avoided or kept to a minimum. Found in butter, lard, cheese, full-fat milk, cream and meat, too much of these hard fats will clog up arteries, block the lymph system that gets rid of waste matter, and cause dull, unhealthy skin.

Monounsaturates and polyunsaturates are good for us and contain essential fatty acids (EFAs) which keep skin moisturised from the inside, thus helping to keep it younger looking for longer. These types of fats are usually liquid – vegetable oils and fish oils. Polyunsaturates are also found in sunflower margarine, low-fat spreads and processed foods. This process of hardening the fats, called hydrogenisation, changes their chemical structure so they behave like saturates, the bad fats. But not all margarines and spreads contain hydrogenated fats – check the label before you buy. Another potential hazard from polyunsaturates is that they break down when heated and produce peroxides which encourage free-radical activity. So don't use sunflower or safflower oils or margarines for cooking. A much healthier alternative is a monounsaturate such as olive oil, which remains stable when heated and is ideal for all types of cooking.

Essential fatty acids work by strengthening the delicate membrane that surrounds each cell. A deficiency can be fatal, and even mildly low levels can result in dry skin which ages more quickly. There are two types of EFAs, linoleic acid and alpha-linolenic acid. Linoleic acid is found in green vegetables, soya, nuts, plant oils and seeds. Alpha-linolenic acids are found in fish oils, fish and shellfish.

To be of any use, these acids need to be converted into substances the body can work with. Linoleic acid has to be changed into gamma-linolenic acid (GLA), which is particularly important for healthy skin. However, this process can become blocked by factors such as stress, pollution, infection, alcohol, saturated fats and drugs. A good way of ensuring your body has sufficient GLA is to take a supplement which contains it such as evening primrose oil or borage oil. GLA helps to strengthen our skin from the inside, increasing the moisture content of cells and speeding up the rejuvenation process. GLA is also important for the creation of prostaglandins, hormone-like substances which control every cell and organ of the body.

The alpha-linolenic acids, found mainly in fish oils, are important for the skin as well as being very good for the heart. They contain two important ingredients, eicosapentaenoic acid (EPA), which gets converted into prostaglandins, and docosahexaenoic acid (DHA) which regulates their activity.

Lecithin

Another important nutrient for preserving skin is lecithin, also found in plant oils. Neither a vitamin nor a mineral, it contains both types of nutrients in addition to linoleic acid. It plays an important part in the natural moisturising factors (NMFs) which are found in our skin. These work by moisturising skin from the inside, absorbing and keeping moisture within the skin. It is a common ingredient in skin creams, but is far more effective when taken internally.

Lecithin is good for skin because it helps to remove the build-up of saturated fats that can lead to skin problems. By unblocking the dermis of these fats, it leads to a smoother, clearer complexion. Good sources are unrefined vegetable oils, wheatgerm, soya beans, peanuts, corn, oats and rice.

Other Useful Foods

All oily fish, particularly sardines, are good for your skin because of the high levels of EFAs they contain. These help to stimulate cell renewal and so strengthen skin. The American doctor Benjamin Frank, who has written several important papers on nucleic acids, claims that a diet rich in these foods can help soften lines and increase the skin's natural moisture content.

A very nourishing food, and one that is especially good for skin, is sprouted grains and seeds. Sprouting increases the vitamin, mineral and enzyme levels dramatically and releases important amino acids that improve the quality of protein and neutralise the agents which can impair zinc and calcium absorption. The method is similar to that of sprouting alfalfa seeds (see page 45).

To sprout grains you need a large jam jar, cloth or a piece of muslin and an elastic band. Place a handful of pulses or seeds in the bottom of the jar, cover the jar with the cloth and hold in place with the elastic band. Run cold water into the jar, turn it upside down and drain the water away. This should be repeated several times a day until shoots have appeared.

Herbs are powerful antioxidants and are thought to help prevent premature ageing thanks to their high levels of EFAs in their aromatic oils. A particularly good one is thyme, though all kinds of herbs are beneficial. Although all forms are nutritious, fresh is best. Parsley is an excellent source of vitamin C, even in tiny quantities. Cook with herbs or sprinkle on food whenever you can.

Green tea is also a surprising antioxidant and thought to be helpful to skin. Some skincare companies are investigating the use of it topically in anti-ageing creams, but for now it seems that the occasional cuppa is no bad thing (preferably a low-caffeine variety such as Luaka).

The Role of Supplements

The best way to get your daily 'fix' of vitamins and minerals is by eating the right foods, since the nutrients are synergistic, and are slowly released into our system as required. The arguments against relying on our food sources are first that the use of pesticides and food refining and processing destroy many of these valuable nutrients before they have a chance to work, and secondly that because of our modern, busy lifestyles it's very difficult to ensure our diet contains all the vitamins, minerals and trace elements we need every day. In particular, vitamin E is hard to find in high enough levels from food alone, so a natural source supplement may be a good idea.

Taking supplements in moderation will do you plenty of good and no harm, since few vitamin overdoses are dangerous (very large doses of A and D being the exceptions). Your body simply excretes what it doesn't need.

You can buy specially prepared 'skin supplements' and these should be carefully formulated and include the nutrients listed in this chapter.

Liquid Assets

Some 70 percent of our body weight consists of water, and without it the body cannot metabolise the nutrients it needs. It is vital for getting rid of waste and toxins from the body and for cell renewal. It is quite simply essential for life.

Without sufficient water skin will dry out and become prone to wrinkling, since water is essential to keep moisture levels high in skin cells. The recommended daily amount is six to eight glasses.

The best type of water to drink is filtered tap water. While tap water alone can contain metals such as aluminium and lead and chemicals such as chlorine and fluoride, filtering it will ensure the water you drink is pure. There are now many types of bottled water to choose from, but if you do buy this, make sure it has a low sodium (salt) content. Too much sodium will only dehydrate you. Some bottled waters are also relatively high in nitrates, so check the analysis label before buying. Drinking fresh fruit and vegetable juices is an excellent way to maintain your intake of antioxidants and minerals. Raw fruit juices are packed full of nutrients including enzymes, which are easily destroyed by heat and light. This is why the best way to drink juices is freshly squeezed from the fruit or vegetable to ensure purity and optimum benefits.

A Daily Supplement for Youthful Skin

* Moisturise your skin from the inside with one table-spoon of unrefined, uncooked vegetable oil such as olive oil, sunflower or safflower. Use as salad dressing, in sauces, or drizzled over pasta or potatoes instead of butter.

* Aim to eat 5–15mg of the antioxidant beta-carotene, found in brightly coloured fruit and vegetables such as carrots, green peppers, oranges and apricots.

100G FRUIT OR VEGETABLE	BETA-CAROTENE CONTENT IN MILLIGRAMS
boiled carrots	7.5
red peppers	3.84
apricots	0.4
mangoes	1.8
melons	1
star fruit	1.8

* Include plenty of foods containing the B-complex vitamins, which help to repair skin. These include wheatgerm, rice, oily fish and dairy products.

* Eat at least 70mg of the antioxidant vitamin C, found in fruits such as cherries, blackcurrants, oranges and lemons. Smokers and passive smokers will need extra daily vitamin C supplies.

100G FRUIT OR VEGETABLE	VITAMIN C IN MILLIGRAMS
oranges	54
blackcurrants	200
grapefruit	36
strawberries	77

* Ensure optimum levels of EFAs found in vitamin E and lecithin with unrefined vegetable oils and oily fish. A supplement of evening primrose oil or borage oil may be beneficial.

* Avoid dehydrating drinks such as alcohol and stimulants such as tea and coffee. Instead drink at least 1 litre of pure, filtered water and a glass or two of freshly squeezed fruit or vegetable juice daily.

4

Effective Skincare

As we get older, we tend to panic-buy skincare products. Spurred on by promising advertisements, we impatiently try one new product after another in a quest for our ultimate goal – the wrinkle eraser. We are often disappointed. The wrinkles remain, we're financially worse off and may even end up with new skin problems such as clogged pores, spots and sensitive skin.

By middle age, the average American woman is using some fifteen to twenty different products on her skin every day, adding up to a massive 200 or so chemical ingredients. While we in Britain are not quite so zealous, it's worth bearing in mind as you try yet another new product on your skin that you might not be doing yourself any favours.

Good-looking skin doesn't mean skin that is totally free from lines or wrinkles of any sort. A lived-in, but well-cared-for face is very attractive. Many skincare and cosmetic companies have woken up to the facts that the number of women over the age of thirty-five is rising, and that people generally live longer, but still want to retain their looks. They have responded to this new market by ditching the patronising advertisements of twenty-year-old models promoting anti-ageing products and instead are playing up the qualities of the older model. Think of Isabella Rossellini, Lauren Hutton and Catherine Deneuve – all well over thirty-five, they are role models to whom older women can relate. Their message is no longer that to be beautiful you have to be young, but that beauty evolves with age.

There is no big secret to healthy, young-looking skin. Once you've nourished it effectively from the inside, skin will respond well to a simple but regular skincare routine. There are just two essential steps for any routine: cleansing and moisturising. Anything more than this is optional. Your routine should not be lengthy and time consuming – if it is then you'll often be tempted to skip it. Just five minutes, morning and evening, are all it should take to look after your skin properly.

With the exception of tretinoin (Retin-A) there are no ingredients which will reverse wrinkles, and this one bears the price of extreme sensitivity to sunlight after use. So don't go shopping for a miracle cure in a jar, because there simply isn't one. Instead, look for products which suit your skin type and your budget and stick with them. Any product you use will take a couple of months to establish itself and show any results on your skin, so give it time.

Know Your Skin Type

Skin is a living organ which changes over the years and with the seasons. Its condition is determined by many factors, including weather, pollution, central heating, hormones and stress. In cold, dry weather you may notice your skin feels drier and perhaps irritated, while in summer humidity levels rise causing skin to become oilier. It's unusual for skin to stay true to one type throughout your lifetime, so don't be surprised if it doesn't behave in the same way as it did twenty years ago. Before you can reassess your skincare routine, or start one, if you don't use skincare products at present, take a moment to check your skin type. (Don't confuse these types of skin condition with the genetic skin types discussed on page 27 in relation to sun protection factors.)

Determining your current skin type depends almost solely on the level of sebum (oil) which your skin produces. Basically, the more sebum there is, the oilier your skin will be. Try one of the following methods to determine your skin type:

* Before you wash your face in the morning, press a tissue against your face, holding it in place for a few moments. Hold the tissue up to the light. If completely clean, your skin is dry and possibly sensitive; if there is a slight imprint of sebum, your skin is normal; if there is a clear T-shaped imprint of sebum from the nose and forehead, you have a combination skin type; a complete face imprint signifies an oily complexion.

* Take a magnifying mirror and examine your face in a bright light. Very fine pores, dull texture, dryness and signs of ageing signify a dry or mature skin type. Even-sized, small pores with no spots or dryness show a normal skin type. Visible pores on nose and chin, with a shiny panel on the nose and forehead indicate a combination skin type. Enlarged pores and a shiny, sallow complexion, acne or spots, with only a few lines or wrinkles signify oily skin.

Dry and Mature Skin

This skin type is more prone to premature ageing. Mature skin loses moisture more rapidly as the natural barrier breaks down as we get older. The rate of cell turnover slows down, and so the stratum corneum is replaced less frequently and the cells on the surface remain there for longer. 'Skin dryness is caused by a lack of water in the paper-thin, non-living top layer of the skin, the stratum corneum. Dryness does not affect the deeper layers of the skin, the epidermis and the dermis,' says American dermatologist Dr Thomas Goodman. The point he is making is that, despite what advertisers say, only the top layer of your skin needs moisturising – the lower layers are inside the body, bathed in tissue fluids, and so are never dry. So beware of creams that claim to moisturise the deepest levels of your skin. Bear in mind that the signs of ageing due to dry skin probably won't show up until your fifties – any wrinkling before that will be due to sun damage.

SKINCARE ROUTINE
Cleansing

To help preserve the protective film which covers the stratum corneum (upper layer of the skin) and locks in moisture, avoid using soap and water to cleanse your face as this will only strip it further of moisture. This is because soap is alkaline, whereas the skin is naturally slightly acidic, with a pH of 5.5–6.0. If you prefer wash-off cleansers use a soap-free bar or facial wash, but only use in the morning. Constant wetting and drying of the skin can worsen dryness. But better still, use a cream or oil-based cleanser morning and evening. Apply a little to the skin, massage in gently, leave for a few seconds, then wipe off with cotton wool, a damp flannel or a soft muslin cloth. Tissues are best avoided as they can scratch delicate skins. Toners are not really necessary for your skin type, but if you can't live without one, make sure it's alcohol-free and enriched with useful skin-nourishing extracts.

Moisturising

An essential for all skin types, dry and mature skins need even more moisturising. Best applied immediately after cleansing, choose a moisturiser that absorbs into the skin easily and doesn't leave a greasy film on your face. A richer product can be used at night-time as the skin undertakes much of its renewal process while we sleep. Top up your moisture levels throughout the day, especially in dry environments, by spritzing skin frequently with a water spray or spray-on facial tonic. If your skin is very dry, it may also be worth investing in a humidifier to boost the moisture content of the air.

Combination Skin

This is a very common skin type, even among older women. It reflects the different elements that can affect your skin: oily areas on the forehead, nose and chin may be aggravated by hormonal factors or a diet too rich in saturated fats; dry cheeks are a result of living in dry conditions (central heating, air conditioning), or perhaps a cleansing routine that is too harsh.

Many mistake the dry, flaky patches on nose and forehead for dry skin, when in fact the opposite is true. A condition called seborrhoeic dermatitis, caused by excessive sebum production or hormonal changes, causes the top layer of the skin to flake off. It can also be caused by too much moisturising and inadequate skin cleansing. Treat these patches by cleansing thoroughly with an oil-based cleanser and follow with a very light, vitamin-enriched moisturiser.

Skincare routine
Cleansing
To prevent spots and blackheads, which commonly appear in the oily areas, cleanse twice daily with a soap-free or oil-based cream cleanser. Oil-based cleansers work well on oilier skins as they dissolve the skin's own sebum and gently remove any excess. Toner is not essential, but may help minimise large pores. Use an alcohol-free variety. If you do have spots, avoid squeezing or touching them as this will only spread the infection.

Moisturising

All skin types benefit from moisturising, not just dry types. Apply twice daily after cleansing all over your face, not just the dry bits, as the dehydration that leads to wrinkling is caused not by oil on the skin but by a lack of water in the stratum corneum. The sebum on your skin serves to trap the moisture below this layer.

Oily Skin

Oily skin is not just a teenage problem, it can affect men and women of all ages. Proper cleansing is essential to keep pores unclogged, but excessive cleansing can cause the skin to react by producing even more sebum, so don't overdo it.

SKINCARE ROUTINE
Cleansing

Strange though this may sound, the best type of cleanser for your skin type is an oil-based one, since sebum dissolves in oil, not water. Apply to the skin twice daily, massaging in then removing with dampened cotton wool. For treating spots, tea tree oil is excellent. Dab the neat oil on sparingly with a fresh cotton bud for each blemish.

Moisturising

Just because your skin is oily doesn't mean you don't need a moisturiser. Choose a light one and apply after cleansing. Good quality moisturisers often contain other useful ingredients such as vitamins, sunscreens and herbal extracts which can be helpful for oilier complexions.

Normal Skin

If you're lucky enough to have normal skin, then your main concern is to keep it that way by regular cleansing and moisturising. Cleansing the face with a soft muslin cloth rinsed in water may be all you need in the morning, and you should choose an oil-based cleanser to remove make-up and general grime in the evening. Moisturise skin after cleansing with a light-weight moisturiser that contains vitamins and naturally active herbal extracts.

Exfoliation

In moderation, exfoliants are a good way of keeping skin looking younger by their action of sloughing off the skin's top layer of dead cells. But be careful not to be too vigorous, since the stratum corneum is our first line of defence against harmful elements such as sunlight and pollution. If you like the feel of skin scrubs, choose one with a gentle action, containing very fine abrasive particles, and use just once a week. Alternatively, simply use a soft muslin cloth to buff away flakes of dead skin and dislodge dingy skin cells.

What's in the Bottles?

It's rare these days, particularly at the expensive end of the range, to see a new skincare product that doesn't contain 'special' ingredients that claim to improve the condition of our skin. And it's all too easy to be taken in by promising claims if we don't understand the technology. From 1997, all manufacturers will be legally bound to list all ingredients on the packs, which should help get rid of some of the hype. This is a particularly good idea if you know you're allergic to a certain ingredient – it will be easier to avoid in future. Most reputable manufacturers will be introducing comprehensive ingredients listings well before this date. Here are some of the most commonly used ingredients in anti-ageing products, and what they can – and can't – do for your skin.

Aloe vera is a succulent African plant which was reputed to have been used by Cleopatra as a skin cleanser. It is both a potent natural healer for minor skin problems and even burns and a great skin soother.

Alpha-hydroxy acids (AHAs) are natural acids which are found in fruit, vegetables and protein sources such as milk. The most commonly used AHAs in anti-ageing products are lactic (from milk), malic (from apples), glycolic (from sugar cane) and pyruvic (from papaya). AHAs basically act as a rapid exfoliant, loosening dead skin cells from the skin's surface by dissolving the natural glue-like protein substance which binds these cells together, causing the skin to renew itself faster than it would naturally. Once the old cells have been removed, fresh, new skin cells are exposed which can give the skin a smoother appearance. Skin can look brighter and feel firmer.

Some manufacturers claim that AHAs can work wonders with acne and hyper-pigmentation. AHAs are thought to be particularly useful for those with oily skin as the dissolving effect regulates the flow of the skin's oil. AHAs may also boost the natural production of the moisturising agent, hyaluronic acid, and promote collagen synthesis, although there have been no independent clinical trials to support this as yet. Older, dryer skins may also benefit from using AHAs through the removal of dry, flaky patches on the skin's surface, making the skin more receptive to moisturisers. Many do-it-yourself suntan lotions also contain fruit acids to help the active ingredient, DHA, by loosening the dead skin cells which could block the staining action. Cosmetic products contain between 1 percent and 10 percent AHA, with the lowest obviously being the least effective. The disadvantage is that low levels of AHAs may have no effect, but high levels can be extremely irritating. Any AHA cream should be used with caution and · discontinued should sensitivity occur. AHAs are acids after all, and so it is not surprising that those with sensitive skin may experience a slight tingling or redness after applying creams which contain them. If your skin becomes seriously inflamed or irritated then you should stop using the product immediately. Many of the creams containing AHAs are expensive so it is worth while trying a test sample (if available) before splashing out on a whole bottle.

At the moment, AHAs are classed as cosmetics as it is only their action on the skin's surface which has so far been recognised. Should the rumours that these fruit acids are able to stimulate the production of collagen and elastin be substantiated, then AHAs may become prescription-only 'drugs' like Retin-A (tretinoin).

In beauty salons, AHAs are used in chemical peeling treatments which literally burn off the top layer of the skin (see page 78).

Antioxidants (vitamins A, C, E) are said to work on the skin surface in much the same way as they work internally, by neutralising harmful free radicals created by sunlight, pollution and cigarette smoke.

The vitamin A derivative retinol is included in anti-ageing products under the pretext of helping repair damaged skin. However, this is not an antioxidant – only the vegetable form of vitamin A called beta-carotene has this capacity. Look for natural beta-carotene rather than synthetic, as it is more powerful at limiting the ageing effects caused by free radicals. Vitamin E is a very common ingredient in moisturisers and anti-ageing creams because of its healing effect on skin and is probably one of the most useful to look for. It is a very effective antioxidant and is often used in sunscreens too. However, look for creams like my own that contain natural, rather than synthetic vitamin E as this is at least one-third more potent.

Vitamin C is notoriously unstable, so difficult to use in skin creams, although some of the newer creams have managed to include it successfully.

Avocado oil is highly nutritious and is a good source of the vitamins A, B, D and E, as well as being rich in lecithin. It is also a good source of the essential fatty acid linoleic acid, which strengthens the membranes surrounding the skin cells and contains as yet unidentified substances that have been shown to help regenerate skin cells. Avocado oil is one of the best oils for soothing dry, parched skin.

Beta glucan is derived from yeast and said to repair sun-damaged skin by stimulating the body's immune system to produce healthy skin. It is claimed to regenerate collagen and elastin and reduce the appearance of wrinkles. Claims are not yet founded.

Calendula oil is extracted from the petals of marigolds by steeping them for a fortnight in natural vegetable oil such as almond or olive oil. The extracted calendula oil contains natural steroid substances called sterols and is especially good for treating skin conditions like eczema, or where the skin has been damaged by steroid abuse.

Ceramides are lipids naturally present in the skin's own sebum that help to form a water-resistant seal over the stratum corneum. Creams containing ceramides claim to reinforce the skin's moisture barrier and improve its appearance. They are good moisturisers.

Chamomile is renowned for its anti-inflammatory and skin soothing properties. The secret of the plant's success are substances called azulenes. German chamomile also contains another extract called alpha-bisabolol. Clinical trials at the University of Bonn in Germany have shown that alpha-bisabolol helps repair sun damaged and chemically injured skin tissues. German chamomile is often used in natural skincare preparations like my own for its uniquely soothing action on the skin.

Collagen is what gives skin its structure, and it is implied that by including this common ingredient in anti-ageing creams, it will replenish your own skin's dwindling supply. In fact it is impossible for the collagen molecule to reach the dermis, since it is much too large (except by injections, see page 79). The collagen used in skin creams is extracted from cow hide, and what it does is to help hold water in the skin by forming a gel-like film on the surface, giving it a smoother, firmer feeling.

Cornflower extracts are used in some natural skincare products because of its mildly antibiotic properties which help to soothe the skin. Cornflower lotions are specially soothing for the sensitive area around the eyes.

Echinacea or coneflower is famed for its skin saving properties. Independent clinical studies show that echinacea promotes skin cell regeneration and actively encourages the production of fibroblasts, which eventually form the supporting structure of the skin. Echinacea is also anti-inflammatory and is renowned amongst herbalists for its ability to treat skin disorders such as acne, eczema and psoriasis.

Elastin, like collagen, is included in skin creams to help reinforce our own supplies. But again, the molecules cannot penetrate to the lowest layers of the skin. Extracted from cow fat, it is a good moisturiser.

Essential fatty acids (EFAs), namely gamma-linolenic and linoleic acid, are vital components of all cell membranes and important for the production of prostaglandins, which play a vital role in keeping skin healthy. Although best taken internally (as vegetable oils, evening primrose oil or borage oil), when applied directly to the skin they help to stem water loss.

Eucalyptus essential oil is antibacterial and is used to gently cleanse and purify the skin. The oil is also anti-inflammatory and is excellent for healing spots, boils and pimples.

Eyebright is a herbal extract that is renowned for its ability to reduce puffiness around the eyes. It also helps to clear the eyes themselves, so is sometimes found in eye make-up removers and eye creams.

Hops extract has a soothing and calming effect on the skin, moisturising and skin strengthening properties and can help promote healthy cell growth. It can be found in some naturally active skincare ranges like my own.

Hyaluronic acid is one of the natural moisturising factors (NMFs) found naturally in the lowest levels of the dermis, where it forms part of the tissue that surrounds the collagen and elastin fibres. Able to hold up to 200 times its own weight in water, it makes an excellent moisturiser. Because of this it has a smoothing action on the skin and it is a useful ingredient in many brands of skin creams.

Liposomes first appeared in the Eighties and were heralded a major breakthrough, allowing active ingredients to penetrate deeper into the skin by 'carrying' them to their destiny, then slowly releasing them. Liposomes are tiny bubbles made up of a lipid (fatty) layer and a water layer, then filled with an active ingredient. There is some evidence that liposomes can give longer-lasting moisturising effects due to their slow-release action, but there is controversy over whether they can penetrate the epidermis or upper levels of the skin. Nanospheres are simply a smaller version of liposomes, claimed to penetrate deeper into the skin thanks to their small size.

Panthenol is the stable form of panthothenic acid which is a B complex vitamin necessary for the normal functioning of the skin. Panthenol moisturises the skin and promotes tissue regeneration and is often used in high quality skincare products.

Phospholipids such as lecithin are found in the cell membrane and help to keep it healthy and watertight. As we age, the phospholipids become depleted, so by adding them to creams, manufacturers claim, the balance is restored. Whether this is true is not well proven, but they do help to make good moisturisers, particularly for older skin.

Rosemary is a herb with invigorating properties and has been used for centuries in beauty preparations. The essential oil has been found to contain a substance called diosmin which helps strengthen fragile capillaries and may even improve disfiguring skin conditions such as broken thread veins. It certainly helps to stimulate, tone and purify the skin.

Wheatgerm oil is another important beauty care ingredient as it is our richest source of the antioxidant and potent skin healer vitamin E. It comes from the seed or 'germ' of the wheat stalk and is also rich in many vitamins and essential fatty acids that strengthen the skin. Wheatgerm is also used as a natural preservative in some skin creams.

Witch hazel is one of the most widely used plants in Western medicine and the leaves contain high levels of a particular tannin, hamamelitannin, which has astringent and anti-inflammatory properties. Witch hazel is often used in skincare preparations to tighten and tone sensitive skin.

Hints on Choosing Skincare

Confronted with row after row of skincare brands, each subdivided into products for particular skin types, shopping for skincare products can be a confusing business.

In Britain we spend some £350 million a year on facial skincare products, and by far the fastest-growing area is anti-ageing products. But while around 70 percent of skincare products bought are moisturisers, relatively few women buy cleansers. Despite advice from dermatologists, as many as 65 percent of women are thought to use soap and water on their face from time to time. Soap is alkaline in nature, and upsets the skin's natural acidic balance, making it feel tight and dry, and it takes a while for the skin to redress the balance. If you're a soap and water addict, turn to the new soap-free cleansing bars instead.

Your first criteria in choosing a product will probably be price. You can pay anything from £1 to £100 for a moisturiser, but is it worth spending a lot? With the more expensive brands you're paying for higher quality ingredients, the technology which created the new 'special' ingredients, the elegant packaging and image and usually a better texture. But in terms of what the product will actually do for your skin, the benefits of using an expensive product are less clear. In recent years the technological advances used in premium brands have been filtering through to the cheaper brands with increasing speed. It's now true that you can get virtually the same benefits from a product costing £10 as one selling for £40. In a consumer study of anti-ageing creams in France, a budget vitamin E anti-wrinkle cream came out top for performance, despite being one of the cheapest brands tested!

Be guided by how the product feels on your skin. A moisturiser should be easily absorbed, not leave a greasy film on your skin. It's a good idea to go for one that gives a longer lasting effect, so you won·t need to keep reapplying. Above all, choose a cream that you are confident contains genuinely high levels of skincaring ingredients. If you find yourself confused by the technological hype of some moisturisers, look for those that are rich in naturally active ingredients such as essential oils and herbal extracts. These skincare ingredients have been tried and tested for centuries and their skin protecting and nourishing properties are well documented. However, beware clever marketing ploys that advertise products are 'natural', when they only contain very low levels of naturally active ingredients. Whether you choose cream, lotion, gel or oil is purely personal although, in general, drier skins should opt for slightly thicker moisturisers, while oily skins should stick with more fluid products.

Cleansers come in an equally confusing number of choices: creams, lotions, rinse-off gels and soap-free bars. You can also buy combined cleansers and toners, which can save you time and money if you like using toner. Soap and water will cleanse off water-soluble dirt, but its alkaline nature can upset the skin's natural pH balance, leaving it dry and tight. It is also not as effective for dissolving oil-based make-up or the skin's own sebum.

The first rule of a cleanser is that it should get rid of all impurities such as oil, grime, make-up and loose dead skin cells with ease. The second is that it shouldn't leave a residue, which can clog up pores and lead to spots. The rest is up to you. In general, wash-off cleansers are best suited to oilier skin types and cream-based to drier skins. If you have sensitive skin, avoid soap, fragrance and colour. One of the best universal cleansers is an oil-based formula, which removes make-up as well as dirt, and suits every skin type, even the sensitive. My own comes with muslin face cloths for swift, effective removal and a gentle exfoliating action.

You may also need a separate eye make-up remover which will remove heavy eye make-up without irritating the eyes. Opt for a gentle formula rich in soothing, anti-inflammatory herbal extracts such as the aptly named eyebright.

Anti-Ageing Extras

EYE CREAMS
The eyes are usually the first area where lines appear and naturally cause concern. In the past few years eye creams have grown from nothing to an important money-spinner – every skincare range now seems to have one. Most claim to hide the appearance of fine lines, reduce puffiness and generally smooth the eye area to make the signs of ageing less noticeable. The basic ingredients of eye creams and moisturisers are the same, though they usually contain more oil to help minimise fine lines. Eye creams may, however, go through more stringent ophthalmic testing to make sure they won't irritate the sensitive eye area. They are also very quickly absorbed and won't leave a greasy film which could make eyes puffy.

FIRMING SERUMS

These are designed to be used occasionally to give skin an instant boost. Basically they are 'super' moisturisers, and by holding water on to the skin's surface they have a temporary firming, plumping and smoothing effect, making your complexion look more radiant and perhaps younger. However, because they are very rich (and expensive too!), keep them for special occasions or use when your skin is in need of a lift. Ingredients include proteins to give a tightening effect, vitamins E and A, silicon, alpha-hydroxy acids, moisturising agents, soothing plant extracts and liposomes.

Night Creams

Night creams are nothing new – women used to put cold cream on their faces before going to bed thirty years ago. The new ones tend to contain more active ingredients than daily moisturisers, since skin is supposedly more receptive and cell renewal is highest when we're resting. They also tend to be richer (or thicker) and this is more acceptable for night-time use. They are not essential, but can be beneficial for drier skin types. If your skin is oily or combination, your normal daytime moisturiser will do just as well. However, the advantage of night creams is that they do not contain unnecessary sunscreens and usually have a higher concentration of useful herbal and vitamin extracts.

— 5 —

Facial Treatments

Looking after your skin doesn't have to cost a fortune and it's ironic that while the skincare industry invests millions in developing new technology, there is a huge interest in naturally based formulas that have been used for decades. For cheaper and more fun alternatives to shop-bought skincare products, why not have a go at making up your own lotions and potions from simple ingredients in your own kitchen? As well as being able to tailor products to meet your individual skincare needs, you'll know exactly what has gone into them too.

DIY Facial Treatments

STEAMING

Begin your DIY skincare routine by thoroughly cleansing the pores, making skin more receptive to moisturisers and masks. As well as deep cleansing, the water in steam will also help to plump up the skin, helping reduce the appearance of fine lines. If you have sensitive skin or broken veins on your face, only use steams occasionally. Steams are good for combination and oily skin types as they help to get rid of blackheads and spots by unblocking clogged sebum from the pores.

Fill a large bowl with just boiled water which has cooled slightly. Add one tablespoon of dried lavender and sage for normal skin; chamomile and basil for dry skin; mint and lemon peel for combination and oily skins. Stir the herbs in and allow to infuse for a few minutes. Place a large towel over your head and neck, forming a tent over you, and lean over the bowl. Close your eyes and allow steam to work on your skin for one–three minutes. Afterwards blot skin dry with a face cloth and spritz with flower water (see page 77).

As an alternative to dried herbs, try a few drops of essential oils added to hot water instead.

For normal skin, use 3 drops lavender, 3 drops mandarin.
For dry skin, use 3 drops rose, 3 drops chamomile.
For combination skin, use 3 drops lavender, 3 drops cypress.
For oily skin, use 3 drops lemon, 3 drops eucalyptus.

EXFOLIANTS

For best results, use your exfoliant after a facial steam. Regular exfoliating will boost the circulation of blood to your face as well as sloughing off the dead skin cells that can give your complexion a dull tinge. This action will speed up the rate by which the skin cells are renewed, encouraging clearer, younger-looking skin to the surface. Regular exfoliation (about twice a week) can help thicken the epidermis, improve dry skin and give better skin tone. Many of the exfoliants or scrubs you can buy are simply too harsh, so try making your own to suit your skin type.

For fragile, dry skin

Take 25g (1oz) ground almonds, 5ml (1tsp) runny honey and one egg white. Grind the almonds in a coffee grinder, then mix with honey to form a sticky paste. Lightly beat the egg white so that it is still liquid, but has doubled in volume. Stir into the almond and honey paste. Apply to clean skin, leave for fifteen–twenty minutes, then massage in using circular movements. Rinse thoroughly.

For all skin types

Take one ripe papaya fruit, slice in half and peel away the skin in large pieces. Rub the inside of the skin over your face and neck, massaging for one–two minutes. Rinse with cool water and pat dry. This treatment works by the enzymatic action of papain found in papaya fruit. Papain dissolves dead keratin, found in dead skin cells.

For dry, dingy-looking skin

Take 15ml (1tbsp) medium ground oatmeal, 30ml (2tbsp) rose water, 1tsp granulated sugar and 1tsp honey. Mix all the ingredients together until they form a gritty paste. Apply to skin using gentle, circular movements, concentrating on the nose, chin and forehead to remove flakes of dry skin. Rinse well and pat skin dry.

For combination skin

Rub fine granules of sea salt into wet skin and massage lightly. Rinse well and pat dry.

For oily or spotty skin

Mix 15ml (1tbsp) granulated white sugar with a few drops of hot water and massage gently over face and neck using circular movements. Rinse with cool water and pat dry. The sugar has an anti-bacterial effect on the skin.

FACIAL MASKS

Masks are the ultimate beauty indulgence and have been used by women for centuries to revitalise their complexions. Used once a week to give your skin a treat, they are simple and quick to make yourself.

For tired, dehydrated skins

Take one small ripe banana, 25g (1oz) finely ground oatmeal and 5ml (1tsp) runny honey. Mash the banana to a smooth paste, stir in oatmeal and honey, and apply to face and neck. Leave on for fifteen–twenty minutes, then rinse off with warm water and pat skin dry.

For dry skin
Give an instant moisture boost with half a ripe avocado, one egg yolk and 5ml (1tsp) olive oil. Mix to a smooth paste and apply to skin. Leave for fifteen–twenty minutes and then remove with damp cotton wool.

For combination or oily skin
Take 10ml (2tsp) Fuller's earth, 10ml (2tsp) witch hazel and one egg white, lightly beaten. Mix the earth with the witch hazel to form a smooth paste, add the egg white and mix in, then apply to nose, chin and forehead with a make-up brush. Leave for five–ten minutes, then rinse thoroughly.

SKIN-FIRMING TREATMENTS
Natural ingredients make excellent skin-firming treatments, with many of these ingredients used in commercially prepared products.

For a skin tightening and brightening effect, mix together 25ml (1oz) witch hazel with 1tsp cider vinegar. Splash the mixture on to skin, then smooth on one lightly beaten egg white. Leave for fifteen minutes, then rinse with cool water.

Make your own AHA treatment to help stimulate cell renewal with this recipe, particularly suitable for mature skins. Dissolve 25g (1oz) brewer's yeast powder in 60ml (4tbsp) freshly pressed apple juice, then stir in 30ml (2tbsp) plain live yoghurt. Apply to face and neck, leave for fifteen minutes, then rinse thoroughly. Lactic acid (found in milk and yoghurt) and malic acid (from apples) are common ingredients of shop-bought AHA creams, while brewer's yeast is thought to encourage skin cells to renew themselves.

Tone and firm up sagging skin with this treatment based on linseeds. Grind 30ml (two level tablespoons) linseeds to split open seeds, then mix with hot water to form a thick paste. Add two drops of cypress essential oil and stir. Spread the mixture on to one half of a piece of muslin or cotton gauze, place on lower half of face, then fold the other half on top to seal. Place a small towel on top to keep in the heat. Leave for ten minutes.

Facial Massage Using Plant Oils and Essential Oils

The use of pure plant oils on the face for cleansing and moisturising goes back to Egyptian times, when oils were prized for their ability to protect and repair the skin. Scientists have yet to improve on nature, and the last few years have seen a surge of interest in these ancient beauty products. Oils make such excellent beauty products because they are compatible with our own sebum, and can help to restore the skin's natural levels of sebum, keeping skin supple and young looking. Oils are suitable for all skin types, including oily, and will not clog pores as is commonly misunderstood, since oil dissolves best in oil.

OILS AND MASSAGE

The best way to use oils on your face is to apply them through massage, which encourages absorption of the oils. Massage helps stimulate your circulation, increasing the oxygen levels in the skin cells, and boosts the lymphatic system which rids the body of waste matter.

Pour a little oil (see below for recommendations) into the palm of your hand, then smooth over face and neck with your fingertips. With your fingertips, tap the skin lightly all over, working from the hairline down, then up again from the throat. Then, use the middle finger of both hands to smooth skin across the forehead, cheeks and chin. Use the back of the fingers to smooth the skin under the chin.

To encourage lymph drainage, take the middle fingertip of each hand and press gently along each eyebrow and around the eye socket, place both fingertips at the corner of the inner eye and smooth skin downwards following the line under each cheekbone. Use thumbs and index fingers to pinch gently along the jawline, starting with the chin and working out towards the ears.

WHICH OILS TO CHOOSE

You can make up your own facial oil blends by combining unrefined 'carrier' plant oils with essential oils. A carrier oil is necessary to disperse the essential oils. Wheatgerm oil is an

ESSENTIAL OILS FOR MASSAGE	
SKIN TYPE	ESSENTIAL OIL
Normal	Basil, chamomile, sandalwood, ylang-ylang, lavender
Dry or sensitive	Chamomile, sandalwood, geranium, neroli
Mature	Rose, patchouli, sandalwood, cypress, geranium, frankincense
Combination	Sandalwood, patchouli, geranium, bay, bergamot, lemon
Oily	Bay, bergamot, juniper, lavender, lemon, eucalyptus

excellent choice as it contains very high levels of the antioxidant vitamin E, helping to guard against ageing. Avocado and hazelnut oils are easily absorbed by the skin and rich in essential fatty acids, while other good choices include jojoba, olive, almond, passionflower, peach nut, apricot kernel, evening primrose and sesame. All can be found in good health-food shops, pharmacies or supermarkets.

There are over 300 types of essential oils, which are extracted from plants and flowers, each with its own therapeutic properties. Because they are so highly concentrated, you will only need a few drops in your blends.

MAKE YOUR OWN BLENDS
For mature skins or those needing a boost
Blend 25ml (1fl oz) jojoba oil with 25ml (1fl oz) wheatgerm oil in a jar, pierce five evening primrose oil capsules and add their contents, together with three drops of frankincense essential oil. Shake thoroughly, then massage into skin using small circular movements. Apply this in the evening and leave on overnight for softer, smoother skin.

For an anti-ageing, firming treatment
Blend 25ml (1fl oz) almond oil, 25ml (1fl oz) jojoba oil, the contents of five evening primrose oil capsules, ten drops of wheatgerm oil, ten drops of frankincense and ten drops of geranium oil. Massage into skin and leave overnight.

For combination skin
Blend 50ml (2fl oz) jojoba oil with ten drops of lavender and ten drops of geranium essential oils. Massage in well and leave overnight.

For oily skin
Blend 50ml (2fl oz) jojoba oil with ten drops of patchouli, five

drops of lemon and five drops of cypress essential oils. Massage in thoroughly.

CLEANSING

Oil blends make good cleansers too, gently dissolving away make-up, grime and excess sebum. Pour the oil into the palms, rub together and then massage all over face. Then take a face flannel wrung out in hot water and wipe away the oil. When all traces of oil are removed, rinse the flannel in cold water and dab over the skin. Keep the flannel washed regularly to avoid infection.

For dry skins

Mix 50ml (2fl oz) almond oil, 50ml (2fl oz) avocado oil and ten drops of rose or sandalwood essential oils.

For normal skins

Blend 50ml (2fl oz) jojoba oil, 50ml (2fl oz) almond oil and ten drops of lavender essential oil.

For combination or oily skin

Mix 100ml (4fl oz) jojoba oil with ten drops of bergamot or mandarin essential oil.

Quick and Easy Youthful Skin Tips

* Enrich your normal moisturiser by piercing an evening primrose oil capsule and mixing in its contents.

* Honey is well known for its skin-healing and moisturising properties. The sugar content is similar to that found naturally in the skin and provides an invisible protective layer on the skin. Give skin a moisture boost

by massaging in two tablespoons of honey, then dip fingers into hot water and massage further. Rinse face clean in tepid water and pat dry.

* Yoghurt and buttermilk contain naturally high levels of the AHA lactic acid, which stimulates the skin to renew itself. It makes an excellent base for a face mask. Try mixing it with grated apple, which contains malic acid, another good alpha-hydroxy acid.

* Soothe puffy eyes and reduce the appearance of fine lines by putting rinsed chamomile tea-bags in the fridge and then placing on to closed eyes for twenty minutes.

* To keep skin well moisturised throughout the day, especially in dry, centrally heated environments, spritz the face frequently with a flower water (remember to close your eyes!). For flower water, fill a pump spray bottle with 100ml (4fl oz) of filtered water mixed with five drops of sandalwood and five drops of rose essential oils. Shake before each spraying and keep in the fridge.

* Water is essential for smooth, supple skin. Drink six to eight glasses of filtered water a day and keep the atmosphere you work in moist by using a humidifier or keeping bowls of water near radiators.

Professional Anti-Ageing Treatments

A certain degree of ageing is natural and inevitable, and how you cope with it is an individual thing. More and more women are not content to accept the signs of ageing and look to science to put things right. The treatments can be expensive, painful and disappointing. If you are considering something stronger than an over-the-counter cream, the key is to do your research first. Find out whether the doctor, dermatologist or beautician is qualified and experienced in carrying out your chosen treatment and speak to other women who have been treated by them. Seek opinions from several sources before you make your choice. One final point to bear in mind: ask yourself why you feel the need to have anti-ageing treatment. 'If people do change their appearance because they want to feel good about themselves, that is fine. If it is going to help their self-esteem and allow them to reframe a situation, they should do it. But they should most definitely not do it because they feel it is what others expect,' says Colin Turner, founder of the Institute of Human Development (UK).

CHEMICAL PEELS

The use of AHAs in creams originates from the chemical peel, which uses high concentrations of these acids to literally peel off layers of skin, revealing younger, smoother skin below. As well as burning off the dead stratum corneum, some of the lower live layers are peeled off too, eliminating fine lines and wrinkles with them. The skin reacts by becoming red and crusting after the peel; this can last for two to three weeks, after which it should heal itself, revealing the younger, softer skin. Chemical peels are painful and should only be carried out by a qualified and experienced surgeon. A bad peel can result in scarring and uneven, patchy-looking skin.

Professor Nicholas Lowe, who runs the Southern California Dermatology and Psoriasis Centre, believes good preparation is essential for a successful peel and to help prevent problems afterwards. His patients are put on retinoic acid therapy for six weeks before the peel, which helps speed up skin renewal after the peel. He has found that peels work best on patients with badly sun-damaged skin, while those with few wrinkles and thin, dry skin tolerate them less well. If you're unsure how your skin will react, you can ask to have a patch test done first. In general, peels are not recommended for women under forty. For best results, you need a series of three or four peels and skin should always be protected with a good sunscreen afterwards.

DERMABRASION

Dermabrasion works on the same principle as chemical peeling, by removing the upper layers of the skin and encouraging the lower layers to grow through smoother and younger looking. Instead of acid to burn away the skin, an instrument is used which strips away the layers of skin. Not quite as effective as peels for erasing wrinkles and lines, it is claimed to be good for removing scars from acne or injury. Risks include pigment problems and scarring.

LASER TREATMENT

A good alternative to surgery in the treatment of age spots and uneven skin pigment caused by ageing, laser therapy is almost painless and leaves little scarring. A series of several sessions will be required. This treatment is only suitable for superficial areas of pigmentation.

LINE-FILLING INJECTIONS

Injections of collagen taken from cow hide to fill out lines and wrinkles have become a very popular alternative to cosmetic surgery in the US, and usage is growing in Britain. However, the effects tend to be short-lived as the new collagen gets quickly broken down and absorbed by the body and injections need to be repeated every few months to maintain the effect.

Before you can have a full collagen injection you will first be tested for sensitivity, since some people are allergic to it. There are three different strengths of collagen used, and the one chosen will depend on where it is to be used and the depth of the wrinkles. The procedure is relatively painless.

A fairly new substance called Fibril is used in a similar way to collagen. Fibril is made up of a gelatin powder mixed with the patient's own blood plasma, which works by stimulating collagen production.

An up and coming method of line filling is lipotransplantation, which is literally the removal of fat from an area of your body such as the thighs or abdomen and injecting it into the face. The problem is that the fat tends to be reabsorbed fairly quickly, giving only short-term results.

Silicone rubber has had a lot of bad press, mainly from its use in breast implants, but used correctly its effects are longer lasting than any other line filler currently available. It is only really suitable for large wrinkles, such as around the nose and mouth. Treatment needs to be carried out gradually and carefully, with at least five sessions, each three to four weeks apart. It is vital that the silicon used is pure and the injections are carried out by an expert, since any mistakes are permanent. Its use is banned in the US because of the problems associated with it, but it is still used in Britain.

FACE LIFTS WITHOUT SURGERY

Electrotherapy is a fairly recent development, offering a cheaper, painless alternative to the scalpel. There are a number of different methods to choose from, but they all work on the basis of applying a mild electric current to the face to stimulate the muscles underneath.

The Perfector treatment uses a computer to transmit tiny microcurrent impulses through the skin to the underlying muscle and tissue. The current is applied to the skin via two hand-held cotton-tipped electrodes, stimulating the specific area being treated. The Perfector lengthens and releases the muscles of the forehead to help reduce tension and frown lines.

It also works on the muscles of the cheeks, chin and throat to tone the underlying muscles and tighten the skin.

The Microlift method is said to boost lymphatic drainage as well as tone sagging skin and can be used on other areas of the body as well as the face. It is claimed to stimulate collagen production.

With Ionithermie, layers of damp muslin soaked in clay are placed on the face on top of treatment creams and two kinds of electric currents applied. The first causes the muscles to contract and relax, and the second encourages deeper absorption of the creams.

Cathiodermie is a very popular method, developed by French chemist René Guinot. A gel-like substance of plant, marine and herb extracts is applied to the skin and massaged in using metal rollers which transmit a mild electric current, helping the gel to penetrate deeper into the skin and stimulating cell renewal. There are several different types of Cathiodermie treatments, depending on which area of the body is being treated. These include anti-ageing treatments for the eye area and neck. However, they should all be avoided by those with fragile and sensitive skins.

SALON FACIALS

Any type of facial treatment you have which involves massage of the face will help improve your lymphatic system, promoting speedy elimination of harmful toxins. Massage will also improve the blood supply to the capillaries in the face, keeping it well hydrated and firmer in tone. The use of acupressure in a facial can also help, as well as being a good stress reliever. Most salon facials also use some form of facial scrub to dislodge dingy skin cells, and a clay-based mask to draw out deeply embedded impurities.

While you can, of course, carry out your own facial at home and learn to use massage techniques on yourself, it is undoubtedly better to have someone properly trained do it for you. As facials are not cheap, why not treat yourself to one occasionally or ask for one as a Christmas or birthday present. Your skin should feel the benefits for at least a couple of weeks afterwards and they are an excellent pick-me-up.

Glossary

Alpha-hydroxy acids (AHAs) – Natural acids found in fruit, milk and sugar which help loosen the bonds between skin cells on the skin's surface, making them fall away faster.

Antioxidant – A substance which prevents oxidation in the cell which leads to free-radical activity and cell damage. Common antioxidants include vitamins A (in the vegetable form of beta-carotene), C and E.

Beta-carotene – Found in brightly coloured vegetables and fruit, the body stores beta-carotene and converts it to vitamin A as needed. A powerful antioxidant.

Collagen – A tough, fibrous protein which makes up the majority of connective tissue in the dermis, giving support and strength to skin.

Dermatologist – A doctor specialising in disorders of the skin.

Dermis – Thick, elastic layer of tissue beneath the epidermis which gives strength and support to skin. Contains blood vessels, hair follicles, sweat glands and sebaceous glands.

Elastin – Protein which forms the elastic fibres in the dermis which keep skin supple and resilient.

Epidermis – Thin layer of living skin below the stratum corneum which produces keratin and contains pigment-forming cells which tan the skin.

Essential fatty acids – A group of unsaturated fatty acids which are vital for healthy growth but cannot be produced by the body so must be supplied by the diet. Commonly found in plant and vegetable oils, such as sunflower, olive and evening primrose oils.

Free radical – A harmful particle, created by oxidation, which causes ageing by damaging the nucleus of our celsl. Free radicals are unstable molecules with an uneven number of electrons that go around stealing electrons from other molecules and causing a chain reaction of cellular damage. They are triggered by sunlight and pollutants such as cigarette smoke and car fumes.

Gamma-linolenic acid (GLA) – A fatty acid naturally found in evening primrose oil and breast milk. It can be produced by the body from linoleic acid and helps increase the moisture content of skin cells.

Hyaluronic acid – Found naturally in the dermis, it forms part of the tissue that surrounds the collagen and elastin fibres. Able to hold up to 200 times its own weight in water, it makes a good moisturising ingredient.

Keratin – Hard protein substance found in skin, hair and nails.

Lecithin – A lipid (fat) which forms an important part of the cell membrane. Found in all vegetable oils.

Linoleic acid – An essential fatty acid found in plant oils, seeds and green vegetables; important for healthy skin.

Liposome – Tiny spheres made up of a fatty layer and a water layer filled with active ingredients and 'carried' to where they are needed in the skin.

Melanin – Skin-colour pigment activated by sunlight which causes a tan.

Monounsaturated fat – Liquid fats from vegetables and plants, such as olive oil, which contain one double-bond. They are stable at high temperatures, resistant to oxidation and believed to be the healthiest type to eat.

Photo-ageing – Wrinkled and sagging skin caused by exposure to sunlight.

Polyunsaturated fat – Liquid fats from plants, vegetable and fish oils, such as sunflower oil, containing two or more double-bonds. The process of hydrogenisation to harden these fats causes them to behave like saturates, while heating at high temperatures produces peroxides. This is why margarines may not be as healthy as they first appear. Many seemingly low-fat, healthy brands of margerine contain hydrogenerated fat which is bad for us.

Prostaglandin – Biological regulators that control the activity of every cell in the body.

Retinoic acid (tretinoin; Retin-A) – The only substance so far that can reverse wrinkles, it is a derivative of vitamin A and was originally prescribed for acne in the 1970s. It speeds up skin-cell renewal and is claimed to boost collagen synthesis. Extreme sensitivity to sunlight, peeling and redness are the drawbacks. It is only available on prescription for the treatment of acne.

Retinol – A type of vitamin A found in animal produce such as liver, milk, eggs, cheese, butter and oily fish. While a certain amount is important, an overdose can be dangerous, particularly for pregnant women.

Saturated fat – Solid fat usually of animal origin such as butter, lard and egg yolks; believed to raise cholesterol levels.

Sebum – An oily substance secreted by the sebaceous glands which keeps skin supple and water resistant and wards off bacteria.

SPF (sun protection factor) – A guide to the effectiveness of sunscreen products. For example, if your skin normally burns after ten minutes in the sun, an SPF8 sunscreen will allow you to stay out for eighty minutes without burning.

Stratum corneum – The layer of dead cells which form the skin surface.

Tocopherol – The medical term for vitamin E, the most important antioxidant, which helps protect skin from premature ageing. Can help repair sun-damaged skin.

UVA, UVB, UVC – Respectively, long, medium and short wavebands of ultraviolet rays from sunlight. UVA is responsible for skin ageing and sun allergies, UVB for burning and skin cancer; UVC rays are filtered out by the ozone layer before they reach the earth.

Useful Addresses

Acne Support Group
16 Dufours Place
Broadwick Street
London W1V 1FE
Send a SAE for information.

The British Association of Aesthetic Plastic Surgeons
Royal College of Surgeons
35–43 Lincoln's Inn Fields
London WC2A 3PN
Tel: 0171 405 0300

Collagen UK Information Service
The Business Centre
6 Bertie Road
Thame OX9 3FR
Tel: 0800 888000

Disfigurement Guidance Centre
PO Box 7
Cupar
Scotland KY15 4PF
Send a SAE for information.

Evening Primrose Oil Office
4 Cupar Road
Battersea
London SW11 4JW
Tel: 0171 720 8596

The International Federation of Aromatherapists
The Department of Continuing Education
Royal Masonic Hospital
Ravenscourt Park
London W6 0TN
Send a SAE for list of local practitioners.

John Bell & Croyden
52–54 Wigmore Street
London W1H 0AU
Stock a wide range of herbal supplements and pharmacy
ingredients. Mail order available.
Tel: 0171 935 5555

Liz Earle Naturally Active Skincare
PO Box 7832
London SW15 6YA
Freephone: 0800 413318

National Eczema Society
163 Eversholt Street
London NW1 1BU
Tel: 0171 388 4097

Play Safe in the Sun Postal Advisory Service
PO Box 4RB
London W1A 4RB

Index